OXFORD MEDICAL PUBLICATIONS

BRITISH PAEDIATRIC ASSOCIATION MANUAL ON INFECTIONS AND IMMUNIZATIONS IN CHILDREN

Steering and writing group:

Dr Peter Rudd (co-editor) *Consultant Paediatrician, Children's Centre, Royal United Hospital, Bath.*

Dr Angus Nicoll (co-editor) *Wellcome Lecturer in the Epidemiology of AIDS, London School of Hygiene & Tropical Medicine.*

Professor Alex Campbell (Convenor) *Professor of Child Health, Royal Aberdeen Children's Hospital.*

Dr Graham Davies *Consultant Paediatrician, Department of Child Health, St George's Hospital, Medical School, London.*

Dr Susan Hall *Consultant Epidemiologist, Communicable Disease Surveillance Centre, London.*

Professor David Hull *Professor of Child Health, Nottingham University Hospital.*

Professor Richard Moxon *Professor of Paediatrics, John Radcliffe Hospital, Oxford.*

Dr David Salisbury *Department of Health.*

Dr Helen Zealley *Community Medicine Specialist, Astley Ainslie Hospital, Edinburgh.*

British Paediatric Association

Manual on Infections and Immunizations in Children

SECOND EDITION

Edited by

Dr PETER RUDD
Consultant Paediatrician
Royal United Hospital, Bath

and

Dr ANGUS NICOLL
Paediatrician and Epidemiologist
Department of Tropical Hygiene,
London School of Hygiene and Tropical Medicine

Oxford New York Tokyo
OXFORD UNIVERSITY PRESS
1991

Oxford University Press, Walton Street, Oxford OX2 6DP

Oxford New York Toronto
Delhi Bombay Calcutta Madras Karachi
Petaling Jaya Singapore Hong Kong Tokyo
Nairobi Dar es Salaam Cape Town
Melbourne Auckland

and associated companies in
Berlin Ibadan

Oxford is a trade mark of Oxford University Press

Published in the United States
by Oxford University Press, New York

British Library Cataloguing in Publication Data

A catalogue record for this book is
available from the British Library

Library of Congress Cataloging in Publication Data

British Paediatric Association manual on infections and immunizations in children / edited by Peter Rudd and Angus Nicoll. – 2nd ed.
(Oxford medical publications)
1. Communicable diseases in children–Handbooks, manuals, etc. 2. Immunization of children–Handbooks, manuals, etc. I. Rudd, Peter. II. Nicoll, Angus. III. British Paediatric Association.
IV. Title: Manual on infections and immunizations in children. V. Series.
[DNLM: 1. Communicable Diseases–in infances & childhood–handbooks.
2. Immunization–in infancy & childhood. WC 39 B862] P.J401.B75 1991
618.92'9–dc20 90–288 15

ISBN 0–19–262118–1 (pbk.)

Set by Latimer Trend & Company Ltd

Printed in Great Britain by
Dotesios Ltd.,
Trowbridge, Wilts

Preface

Any comprehensive programme whose aim is to reduce to a minimum, deaths, damage, and distress caused by infectious diseases will contain a number of approaches. Wherever possible the offending organisms should be banished from our islands. The fall in infection rates from poliomyelitis, tuberculosis, mumps, and measles have been very encouraging. Steps to avoid exposure and to improve the general well-being and sturdiness of our children are also important. There is, however, a limit to how successful these strategies can be, certainly within the forseeable future. Newborn babies, infants, and children will still meet infecting organisms and suffer as a consequence. So it is essential we ensure that as many children as possible benefit from the protection given by vaccines, and that infection when it takes hold is recognized early and treated effectively when antimicrobial agents are available. With the continuing introduction of new vaccines and more effective antimicrobial agents, it is a challenge to us to act responsibly so that children gain most benefit with least risk.

Traditionally in the UK, family practitioners, hospital nurses, and doctors have to be concerned with recognizing infection and giving treatment, whilst medical officers and health visitors have been responsible for vaccination programmes. Such a division of function is no longer appropriate. We must all be aware of the overall strategies and take whatever steps we can to ensure that all the programmes are successful. Family practitioners are now central to vaccination programmes and illness treatment. Children who move with families in the margins of our society need special services and more opportunistic attention. Vaccination and treatment of children with complex or chronic health problems need to be more actively addressed. In the last two examples the hospital services have an important part to play.

The aim of this book is to provide all those involved, family doctors, health visitors, and community and hospital staff, with a simple timely guide to the recognition and treatment of infections and the appropriate use of vaccines. The advice on vaccines is consistent with that given in the DHSS green book on 'Immunisation Against Infectious Diseases'.

Dr Peter Rudd has prepared this second edition in double-quick time. The BPA Immunology and Infectious Diseases Committee and I are most grateful to him for taking on the task.

The first edition was a modest success; we are aware that if it is to become a regular companion for all those involved, it will have to be more 'reader friendly' and 'economic'. We hope we have learnt from our first efforts, and that this second edition will be more widely used. If readers have any suggestions for improvements we would like to hear them.

David Hull
Professor of Child Health,
Queen's Medical Centre, Nottingham NG7 2UH

Acknowledgements

I would like to thank all our paediatric collaborators who wrote sections of this book, particularly Professor Alex Campbell, and Dr Susan Hall. Many medical colleagues and authorities, too numerous to mention, contributed information or made valuable comments. The Communicable Disease Surveillance Centre (CDSC) and the Office of Population Censuses and Surveys (OPCS) in London have provided considerable epidemiological information. I am grateful to Dr Graeme Hamilton, Dr Elizabeth Miller at CDSC, Dr Anna McCormick at OPCS, Ms Gill Jones of the National Congenital Rubella Surveillance programme, Dr Deidre Lewis from the PHLS in Bath, and Dr John Maunder of the Medical Entomology Centre, at the University of Cambridge for their help. C. V. Mosby and Company kindly gave permission for an illustration in *Infectious diseases for children* by S. Krugman and S. L. Katz to be used as a basis for Fig. 2. Mr Graham Doyal and the Vaccination and Immunization Committee of Nottingham Health Authority are the source of Figs 7, 8, and 9. The latter also kindly gave permission for us to use portions of its handbook as a starting point for large parts of the immunization section. The Malaria Reference Laboratory of the London School of Hygiene and Tropical Medicine gave advice on protection against malaria, and the British Medical Journal kindly allowed us to reproduce tables 15 to 21 on malaria. Finally I would like to thank Professor David Hull for his support and encouragement, and Mr Paul Dunn, Secretary of the BPA for his practical advice. I am grateful to the Wessex Regional Health Authority who allowed me time to work on this volume.

Peter Rudd

Contents

Immunization

Practical immunization: Questions and answers

Travel abroad

Appendices

Introduction: how to use this book

This handbook is intended for all primary-care and hospital staff working with children: general practitioners, clinic doctors, paediatricians, health visitors, practice nurses, school nurses and clinic nurses, ward nurses, nursing students, junior doctors, and medical students. As a source of information on infectious diseases and immunization other child-care professionals, health administrators, and parents will also find parts of the text useful.

The text may be read through in its entirety but as a handbook it is designed as a source of information and guidance for the user with a specific problem. There is considerable cross-referencing and some repetition so that the reader does not have to skip around the book excessively.

The first section **Clinical problems** gives general guidance on the diagnosis and management of children with infection: respiratory illness, fever, rash, etc. When a variety of organisms may be the cause (e.g. otitis media) some guidelines on treatment are provided in these pages. However, if a more specific diagnosis is possible the reader is referred on to the second section **Diseases** where the principal childhood infectious diseases are arranged alphabetically. Practical details are given for each concerning epidemiology (including mode of transmission and incubation periods), natural history, and management. Antibiotic dosage is given in Appendix 2 where this is appropriate. When diseases have only recently been recognized (examples are AIDS and Kawasaki disease) they are described in more detail; the same applies for newer immunizations (hepatitis B and MMR).

The third section concerns **Immunization** and describes in alphabetical order the vaccines available for children. This gives details for each vaccine of its efficacy, when it should be given, and the rare occasions when it should be withheld. Also in the section are given the essentials of immunization practice: vaccine handling, consent and medical prescription, and immunization reactions. A section **Practical immunization: questions and answers** covers the specific problems that arise in day-to-day immunization (for example, who gives consent when a child is a ward of court). Because of the increasing amount of international travel there is a section on **Travel abroad** concerning preparing for a trip, and including a sub-section on the management of an ill child recently arrived in the UK, **The child travelling from abroad**.

The appendices give lists of notifiable diseases, anti-microbials, exclusion periods, and immunization schedules, sources of specialist advice, and further reading. There is also a glossary and index.

Inside the front and back covers is some information which may be required frequently (immunizations children should have by key ages, and an immunization checklist) or rapidly (managing anaphylaxis).

All the sections cover the activities of both primary and hospital care. A few of those involving very sick children (e.g. severe croup) or severe diseases (e.g. diphtheria) will only be applicable to hospital. Details of management of these conditions are given for the guidance of hospital staff and as information for community practitioners. This is evident from the text. The bulk of childhood infections are presently managed within the context of primary care and undoubtedly should continue to be so. Some cases of mild or moderate illness will benefit from hospital help or advice. The decision on whether to admit a child is rarely simple and this book does not attempt to provide hard-and-fast rules. Our experience as doctors working both in the community and hospital has convinced us of the importance of communication and discussion in the management of infectious disease. Likewise, a telephone consultation between hospital specialist and community practitioner can frequently resolve even quite difficult immunization problems.

The handbook details single well-tried approaches to most problems of diagnosis and management of infection. However, there are often acceptable alternatives and we would not wish to imply that these should not be used.

August 1990

Angus Nicoll
Peter Rudd
British Paediatric Association

Introduction to the second edition

Two years is a short interval between editions, but much has happened to justify another version of this manual. During 1990, immunization schedules were changed so that immunity to Pertussis could be achieved earlier and the new schedules are included. Certain infections have increased in incidence, or have caught the public eye. There are new sections on listeriosis, cryptosporidiosis, and that on toxoplasmosis has been expanded. To respond to our critics we have added sections on the management of meningitis, as well as joint and bone infections, and the appendix listing antibiotic doses should now be easier to use for the hospital doctor. Modifications have been made to the section on immunization of children with special problems which will help those working in the community.

I have received many suggestions as to how this edition might be improved. I hope that these will continue to reach us so that the third edition is even more relevant to those caring for children.

Finally, I have missed the support of Angus Nicoll, Co-editor of the first edition, and look forward to his return from Tanzania.

Child mortality from infectious diseases in the United Kingdom 1987

(International Classification of Disease Codes)

	0–1 yrs	1–4 yrs	5–9 yrs	Total
All infectious and parasitic disease (001–139)	128	73	29	230
Intestinal infectious disease (001–9)	14	3	1	18
Tuberculosis (010–18)	0	1	0	1
Other bacterial disease (020–41)	86	50	16	152
Diphtheria (032)	0	0	0	0
Whooping cough (033)	2	1	1	4
Meningococcal infection (036)	53	40	9	102
Septicaemia (038)	25	5	6	36
Viral disease (045–79)	23	17	11	51
Viral disease of the nervous system (045–9)	9	6	1	16
Acute polio (045)	0	0	0	0
Chickenpox (052)	2	3	2	7
Herpes simplex (054)	1	2	0	3
Measles (055)	1	1	3	5
Rubella (056)	0	0	0	0
Viral hepatitis (070)	1	2	2	5
Mumps (072)	0	0	0	0
Meningitis (320–2)	40	33	4	77
Acute bronchitis/bronchiolitis (466)	76	15	3	94
Pneumonia (480–6)	134	36	11	181
Infections specific to the perinatal period (771)	14	1	0	15

* Excludes deaths during the first 28 days of life in England, Wales, and Northern Ireland.

By courtesy of Office of Population Censuses and Surveys (OPCS): General Register Office (Scotland), and General Register Office (Northern Ireland).

Child infectious disease morbidity

Notifications of disease (in 1988; England and Wales only)

	All ages	0–4 yrs	5–14 yrs
Cholera	17	2	1
Typhoid	174	19	48
Dysentery	3692	827	663
Food poisoning (formally notified or ascertained by other means)	39 704	6176	3756
Infective jaundice	5062	295	1672
Tuberculosis (all)*	5161	124	253
Tuberculous meningitis	73	7	10
Diphtheria	1	0	1
Whooping cough	5117	3164	1710
Scarlet fever	5949	2095	3013
Acute meningitis	2987	1457	419
meningococcal	1304	670	194
pneumococcal	209	90	15
H. influenzae	436	385	23
viral	490	73	110
Ophthalmia neonatorum	374	374	0
Tetanus	12	0	0
Measles	86 000	41 379	39 478
Polio (acute, paralytic, and non-paralytic)	2	0	0
Malaria	1267	45	142

* Excluding chemoprophylaxis

By courtesy of OPCS and General Register Office (Scotland) and General Register (Northern Ireland).

Diseases ascertained from special reporting schemes

A. National Congenital Rubella Surveillance Programme (NCRSP)

Congenital Rubella Syndrome (Great Britain): 6 cases reported in 1989.

B. British Paediatric Surveillance Unit (United Kingdom and Republic of Ireland)

Confirmed cases reported during 3-year period, January 1987 to December 1989.

AIDS in childhood	16
Neonatal herpes	38
Reyes Syndrome	63
Haemolytic uraemic syndrome	268
Congenital toxoplasmosis*	11

* Reporting started in June 1989 and included 7 cases awaiting serological follow-up for final confirmation.

See Paediatric AIDS Cases Table (p. 41) for most recent data.

Immunization targets

The decision to withold immunization should be taken only after serious consideration of the potential consequences for the individual child and the community.

WHO Expanded Programme on Immunization 1984

Realistic minimum targets

Polio Diphtheria Tetanus Pertussis	90 per cent of all children to have three doses by six months
Measles/mumps/ rubella (MMR)	90 per cent of all children to be immunized by 18 months; vaccine uptake should also be reviewed at school entry
Rubella	No girl should enter the child-bearing years susceptible to rubella

These targets are sufficient for satisfactory herd immunity for some diseases: measles, mumps, and pertussis. However, for individual protection the level of vaccine uptake should be exceeded. All health-care professionals should ensure that these targets are achieved for the children under their care. **Community paediatricians carry a particular responsibility in this respect in their own geographical area.**

Adapted from regional WHO targets for Europe 1984

National immunization uptake* (England only)

Diphtheria, tetanus, and polio	87 per cent
Pertussis	75 per cent
Measles	80 per cent

For the period April 1988–March 1989.
Percentage of child population immunized by their second birthday.

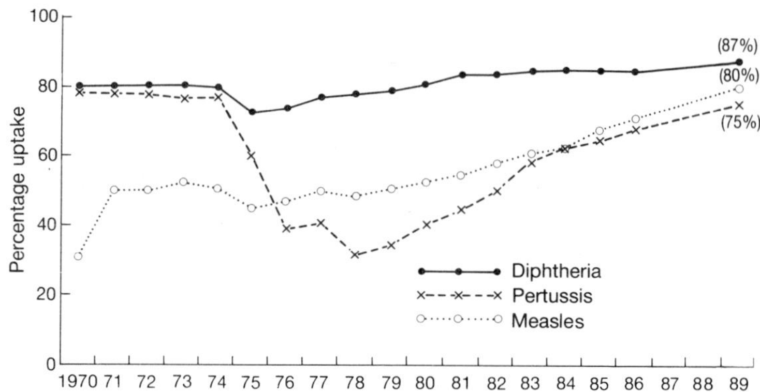

Fig. 1 Immunization uptake in England and Wales 1970–89.
Figures for 1986 and 1989 are for England only. Figures are computed for a year as the number of immunization courses (e.g. three Triples) completed by 31 December of that year for children who were born in the year preceding, divided by the number of live births in the latter year. For example, 1986 figures are all courses completed by 31.12.86 amongst children born in 1984, divided by the number of live births in 1984. The 1989 figures are calculated as described in the national immunization uptake table, above.

The British Paediatric Surveillance Unit (BPSU)

This unit was set up in 1986 on the initiative of the British Paediatric Association to facilitate the surveillance and study of rare childhood infections, infection-related, and other disorders by providing an 'active' case ascertainment facility. It is a joint venture of the British and Irish Paediatric Associations, the Communicable Disease Surveillance Centre, Communicable Diseases (Scotland) Unit, and the Department of Epidemiology of the Institute of Child Health, London.

A report card containing a list of conditions is sent monthly to all hospital consultant paediatricians in the UK and Eire. The reportable conditions involving infection in 1990 are:

- Acquired immunodeficiency syndrome (AIDS) in childhood;
- neonatal herpes;
- subacute sclerosing panencephalitis (SSPE);
- Reye's syndrome;
- Kawasaki disease;
- Rheumatic fever;
- congenital rubella;
- Mumps vaccine induced meningoencephalitis.

For further information contact the Medical Coordinator, BPSU, 5 St. Andrew's Place, London NW1 4LB. Telephone: 071 935 1866.

Clinical problems

Infection in the newborn period and infancy

(Infancy is taken to include the first 12 months of life)

Infection presenting in the neonatal period (the first four weeks of life) may have arisen from invasion by micro-organisms in any one of three periods. First, when *in utero* (congenital); secondly, during labour and passage through the birth canal; thirdly, after birth. Some organisms only infect the baby during one of these periods: examples are rubella *in utero* and respiratory syncytial virus (RSV) after birth. Some bacteria may cause infection during more than one of these periods, as is the case with *Streptococcus agalactiae* (group B). A single micro-organism may produce different signs of infection in the infant depending on the period in which it is acquired. For instance, congenital cytomegalovirus (CMV) may result in deafness and microcephaly but postnatally acquired infection in the term infant is generally mild.

The early signs of infection in the neonatal period and early infancy can be subtle and may include only one or two of those given in the following list: pyrexia, low temperature (rectal temperature less than 36.5°C), irritability, floppiness, tachypnoea, apnoea, loss of interest in feeds, disturbance of the normal sleeping pattern. Young infants showing any of these signs may need hospital referral and should not be prescribed antibiotics as this may mask serious infection and complicate diagnosis.

If a doctor is asked to see an infant after the first month with features including fever and nasal discharge, by far the commonest cause is a viral upper-respiratory-tract infection such as coryza. Parents should be asked about the infant's behaviour. Irritability or difficulty in feeding associated with drowsiness may be signs of more serious infection. The doctor should check carefully for a focus of infection, paying particular attention to the ears, nose and throat, and the respiratory rate. The infant should be undressed completely and examined for evidence of a rash, such as is seen with meningococcal infection. Where the doctor is satisfied that the child does not require hospital admission, it may be useful to leave written instructions for the parents. Some practitioners or community services produce printed cards. An example is:

Check the temperature. If over 38° C but your child is not getting iller then keep the room cool; remove most clothing; give some paracetamol (not aspirin); check your child every 4 hours during the night; **if your child shows any of the following**, phone . . . immediately:

crying, which you cannot stop by comforting, for more than two hours;
very rapid breathing (more than 60/min) while the child is quiet;
a fit or convulsion;
sleepiness or drowsiness that is not a natural sleep;
a rash with what appear to be blood spots in the skin.

Parents may need to be instructed in how to take a temperature using a conventional thermometer under their child's arm. Many will not have a mercury thermometer at home. They should be encouraged to buy one and dissuaded from purchasing a 'strip' surface thermometer as these frequently underestimate body temperature.

Where the diagnosis is unclear but home management appropriate, the doctor should arrange to check the young febrile infant at a later time. If a focus of infection is found to account for the fever it may be appropriate to start an antibiotic; but some arrangements for follow-up must be made to assess the response to treatment. Nevertheless, indications for antibiotic treatment in infancy are few and inappropriate use of these agents—e.g. where there is a possibility, rather than certainty, that otitis media is present, is not recommended. Such treatment may mask meningitis or prevent diagnosis of urinary-tract infection with serious consequences. An exception is where meningococcal disease is suspected. In this case (see p. 90) injection with penicillin may be given prior to transfer to hospital. Unfortunately, the signs of meningitis during infancy are non-specific and can involve changes in the behaviour of the infant, as described above for the neonate. Meningism (a stiff neck) may not occur before 18 months of age; if it does occur early in infancy, it usually implies advanced infection. Also, by 18 months the fontanelle is frequently too small for detection of increased intra-cranial pressure. Because it is difficult to distinguish a febrile convulsion due to meningitis from one associated with a simple virus infection, many paediatricians recommend a lumbar puncture in all infants with a convulsion.

Infants with untreated bacterial infection—meningitis, urinary-tract infection or pneumonia—may deteriorate rapidly and should be referred to a paediatrician where these conditions are suspected. Where the doctor is concerned that the family will be unable to respond to a deterioration should it occur, admission may be justified. If the infant is not admitted to hospital, careful reassessment must be performed in a few hours as circumstances allow. Failure to follow up and check on the non-specific 'warning signals' of infection in infancy is an important error of omission.

The child with respiratory infection

Epidemiology

Infection predominates in any general practice and by far the commonest diagnoses made during childhood are respiratory infections, the common cold, febrile sore throat, and otitis media. Studies of hospital admission rates and patient bed days also show the prominence of respiratory infections and asthma, especially during winter and early spring. Many infections are minor and self-limiting; however, some may represent the early stages of more serious conditions and an important task is to identify these occasional children out of the many who are seen with respiratory symptoms.

Various parts of the respiratory tract may become infected by an enormous range of organisms: viruses, bacteria, chlamydia, mycoplasma species, and fungi. Some infections are responsive to antibiotic therapy which occasionally may be life-saving, but most are caused by viruses and are not susceptible. Thus, it is important to be as precise as possible in diagnosis to ensure early and effective treatment with antibiotics, while avoiding indiscriminate prescribing. The main sites of respiratory infection with the most important etiological agents to be identified are shown in Table 1.

Table 1 Causes and usual treatment of the main respiratory-tract infections

	Principal agents to be considered	Treatment
Common cold	rhinoviruses and adenoviruses	
Influenza	influenza viruses	
Pharyngitis/ tonsillitis	*Streptococcus pyogenes* group A (β haemolytic streptococcus) EBV, adenoviruses	penicillin, amoxycillin amoxycillin and clavulanic acid (augmentin)
Otitis media	*Haemophilus influenzae* *S. pneumoniae* (pneumococcus) adenoviruses	augmentin or amoxycillin (some *H. influenzae* strains resistant to amoxycillin)
Epiglottitis	*H. influenzae* type b	intubation chloramphenicol cefuroxime
Tracheitis	*H. influenzae* type b *Staphylococcus aureus*	intubation cefuroxime and flucloxacillin
Severe croup	para-influenzae viruses	symptomatic ± intubation
Acute bronchiolitis	respiratory syncytial virus (RSV)	hydration tube-feeding physiotherapy
Pneumonias	viruses bacteria *Chlamydia trachomatis psittaci* *Mycoplasma pneumoniae* *Mycobacterium tuberculosis*	initially, penicillin or ampicillin/flucloxacillin. Modify later if specific aetiology identified

Nasal passages: the common cold (coryza)

Most children have several colds each year, especially during the winter months, and some never seem to be free from nasal catarrh and a barking cough. When associated allergies and asthma are present their differentiation from an infection may be difficult. During acute episodes of coryza a profuse watery, later purulent nasal discharge is associated with nasal obstruction and mild constitutional symptoms. A blocked nose is particularly troublesome for infants under six months and complicates breathing and feeding. This may be relieved before feeds by gentle nasal cleansing. Short-term relief can also be obtained by nasal decongestants (Otrivine) instilled just before feeding. Paracetamol will relieve constitutional symptoms and reduce irritability. As these infections are caused by rhinoviruses, antibiotics are not indicated and their early use may mask the development of more serious infection and so delay diagnosis.

Pharyngitis and tonsillitis

A febrile illness with a painful, red and inflamed throat and associated lymphadenopathy is common in childhood especially in the early school years. Many of these infections are viral in origin but the main point of diagnostic importance is to identify the presence of group A beta haemolytic streptococci which may initiate the immune complex diseases: glomerulonephritis and rheumatic fever. Bacterial infection is suggested by a fever and an exudate but viruses such as the Epstein–Barr virus (EBV), the cause of glandular fever, may give an identical appearance, and streptococcal infection does not always cause an exudate. Streptococcal infection needs to be treated with an antibiotic, but this selective policy is only feasible where facilities are available for culture from throat swabs. The antibiotic of choice is oral penicillin V, preferably for 10 days and in severe infections the initial dose, or doses, should be given parenterally as benzyl penicillin.

For all forms of tonsillitis or pharyngitis (viral or bacterial) symptomatic treatment with soothing drinks or gargles and an analgesic such as paracetamol are indicated. An exudative tonsillitis or pharyngitis may be caused by EBV. This diagnosis is more likely where there are characteristic punctate haemorrhages on the soft palate in the mouth.

Otitis media

Ears are a frequent site of acute infection in childhood and a careful ear inspection should be part of every examination. This is particularly true for small infants where localizing symptoms and signs may be absent. Fever, vomiting, irritability, or inconsolable crying are the main clinical features. Older children may complain of painful ears, deafness, headache, or dizziness. Fever can be very high and may precipitate a convulsion. Ear examination can show evidence of an acutely inflamed middle ear with prominent vessels on the tympanic membrane (ear-drum), loss of the light reflex from the membrane, and perhaps some distortion or bulging of the drum. A number of organisms cause otitis media, the commonest being: *Haemophilus influenzae* type b, streptococci, pneumococci, and viruses. A broad-spectrum antibiotic, such as amoxycillin, is indicated for infants and children under three years because of the frequency of *H. influenzae* infection, while penicillin remains the drug of choice for older children. Pain and discomfort should be relieved with paracetamol and decongestants. If clinical exudative otitis media ('glue ear') with associated hearing loss persists, a referral to an ear, nose, and throat surgeon or an audiologist is necessary.

Upper-airway obstruction, croup, and epiglottitis

Mild croup of infancy with noisy breathing during the night and improving by day is relatively common. Apart from a cough and perhaps nasal discharge there is usually only a mild constitutional upset. The child's colour remains normal, there is usually only mild respiratory difficulty when the child is upset, and stridor may be absent at rest. These children can usually be treated at home. However, it is the responsibility of the primary-care physician to recognize that children with persistent stridor can deteriorate quickly, and those with severe respiratory obstruction caused by laryngo-tracheitis and epiglottitis must be transferred to hospital without delay. Indications for hospital admission include stridor at rest, particularly if the preceding history (usually of sore throat and fever) is short and deterioration has been rapid. There may be other signs of marked respiratory distress such as refusal to eat or drink, with drooling of saliva. In severe obstruction the child appears apprehensive and sits upright, leaning forward in a desperate attempt to aid breathing which is becoming increasingly laboured. With this clinical picture, relief of the obstruction is urgently required.

Obstruction of the airway may be caused by viral inflammatory oedema of the sub-glottic airway (laryngotracheobronchitis) or by inflammation of the epiglottis, usually from infection with *H. influenzae* type b. The history and clinical findings may help to differentiate the two. The child with epiglottitis will have a fever, will appear pale, and will frequently drool. The throat of any child with severe obstruction must not be examined anywhere except in the operating theatre or intensive care, nor should he be disturbed by blood tests or X-rays. It is more important to focus attention on protecting the airway from total obstruction which may be fatal and can occur without warning in a child exhausted by the increased effort of maintaining ventilation. Many hospitals have developed policies for responding to this emergency. Treatment of severe obstruction is by urgent intubation performed by an experienced anaesthetist, with an ENT surgeon present where this is possible because, rarely, a tracheostomy will be required. Blood culture and pharyngeal swabs should be taken after intubation and a parenteral antibiotic effective against *H. influenzae* type b (chloramphenicol or cefuroxime) should be given.

If the child's condition is good on admission to hospital and it is agreed that intubation is not required immediately, the child must be nursed where vital signs can be monitored. Frequent (at least half-hourly) observations of colour, heart rate, and respiratory rate, with less frequent measurements of blood gases and pH, will indicate improvement or deterioration within a few hours.

Acute bacterial tracheitis is less common and is caused by *H. influenzae* type b or *Staphylococcus aureus*.

Acute bronchiolitis (see also respiratory syncytial virus p. 98)

This potentially serious infection is common in infants under one year and occurs in epidemics in late winter and early spring. The respiratory syncytial virus (RSV) is responsible for most infections, although other viruses may cause outbreaks. It is a particularly dangerous infection for preterm infants with residual chronic lung disease, and for babies with congenital heart disease and heart failure. Serious outbreaks have been reported from newborn special-care nurseries.

The infection begins like any common cold but a cough, rapid breathing, and wheezing soon develop to the extent that feeding becomes difficult. The characteristic expiratory wheezing results from an inflammatory process causing obstruction of the small airways (bronchioles).

Milder cases show spontaneous improvement after 2–3 days without serious interference with respiration or feeding but in some infants there is progressive breathlessness and cyanosis, continuing hyperinflation of the lungs, widespread moist crepitations, and increasing respiratory acidaemia. Hospitalization is indicated in most such cases, as the baby's condition may deteriorate rapidly and respiratory failure will require assisted ventilation.

RSV can be identified quickly by immunofluorescence of the naso-pharyngeal secretions. This may be helpful in making a decision as to whether antibiotics are required but these may be indicated for a critically ill infant even where RSV has been identified.

General measures in management include tube feeding or even temporary cessation of oral feeding if the infant is critically ill. It is important to maintain adequate hydration if necessary by intravenous infusion.

RIBAVIRIN (VIRAZID), which inhibits a range of DNA and RNA viruses is available for the treatment of severe bronchiolitis, particularly for those infants with chronic lung disease and certain congenital heart defects. It is given by small-particle aerosol for 12–18 hours each day for 3–7 days.

Pneumonia in childhood

Although in bacterial pneumonia the causative agent can usually be isolated from the nose or throat, infection is normally confined to the lung. A lobar pneumonia in the child is, for practical purposes, diagnostic of *Streptococcus pneumoniae* (pneumococcus) infection (see p. 94), although it may be seen rarely with *Staphylococcus aureus* infection (see p. 108). Pneumonia associated with effusion is generally caused by *S. pneumoniae*, and less commonly *S. aureus*. Viral infections of the upper respiratory tract may be associated with pneumonia.

Chlamydia trachomatis pneumonia (see p. 46) should be considered in the young infant, as should bacterial pathogens such as *Streptococcus pneumoniae* (pneumococcus), *Staphylococcus aureus*, and *Haemophilus influenzae* (see p. 67). The bacterial agents are seen throughout childhood, although *Mycoplasma pneumoniae* is unusual under the age of five, while being responsible for up to 20 per cent of cases in school-age children. Tuberculosis must be considered in the differential diagnosis of lower-respiratory-tract infection, especially in recently arrived immigrant children. Immunocompromised children are particularly susceptible to infection with *Pneumocystis carinii* and fungi such as *Candida* sp.

In young children the presentation of pneumonia can be subtle. There may be no obvious respiratory distress, although there will usually be tachypnoea and tachycardia. Added sounds and other clinical findings useful in adults may be absent on auscultation.

The diagnosis should be suspected in infants with fever, grunting, nasal flaring, and tachypnoea, perhaps in association with drowsiness and irritability when disturbed (features suggestive of hypoxaemia). In older children, especially if the pneumonia involves the lower segments of the lung, abdominal pain may be the presenting feature. Right upper-lobe pneumonia can cause neck stiffness without any chest signs and hence masquerade as meningitis.

In almost all circumstances hospitalization is indicated, particularly in infants, as respiratory failure needs to be anticipated and treated. In management, general measures include the provision of humidified oxygen sufficient to maintain adequate oxygenation. If feeding has ceased or is considered dangerous (because of possible aspiration), an intravenous infusion will be necessary to maintain hydration and also provide a convenient access for drugs. Physiotherapy is important where there is extensive consolidation.

Although in many cases a viral aetiology is likely, an antibiotic is usually prescribed, as delay in starting effective therapy can have serious consequences. The pattern of onset, clinical findings, chest X-ray appearances, the leucocyte count and its differential may be helpful in determining the most appropriate antibiotic. When a bacterial pneumonia is suspected, a throat swab and blood cultures should be taken and antibiotic treatment reviewed when the results are available. In early childhood the most likely bacterial pathogens are *S. pneumoniae* and *H. influenzae* type b, but staphylococcal pneumonia should be considered when the initial chest X-ray shows extensive consolidation.

The child with a rash

This section outlines the diagnostic process applied to a child presenting with a rash of rapid onset. Rare causes are not included; the conditions described will, however, cover almost all cases encountered in community practice and in the majority of hospital referrals. Some common rashes of non-infectious aetiology are also included. The management of most of the infectious causes is covered under the named illnesses; however, a few infections are too minor to deserve separate consideration and are covered within this section.

Many rashes look similar and the diagnosis is not based on appearance alone. A history and general examination are essential and a schema for this is as follows.

History

prior infectious diseases and/or rashes,
recent contact with infectious disease,
prior and recent immunizations,
foreign travel,
present and recent medication,
prodromal illness (symptoms appearing prior to rash) especially fever,
similar illnesses occurring in the locality,
itch.

General examination

general state,
temperature,
lymphadenopathy,
splenomegaly,
conjunctivae,
respiratory signs,
signs on the mouth (e.g. Koplik's spots in measles) and ears.

Features of the rash

What form does it take?

Vesicular (fluid-filled sacs);
Maculopapular (a mixture of macules—flat lesions, and papules —raised; as in measles);
Punctiform (pinpoint-like) as in rubella;
Haemorrhagic (petechiae, which are small, or the larger ecchymoses)

Over which part of the body was the rash first seen? What is its present distribution? Is there evidence of scratching?

Rashes in well babies

In community practice healthy young children, and particularly babies, frequently present with trivial punctiform, maculopapular, and even vesicular rashes. During the neonatal period many infants develop an erythematous and sometimes vesicular rash (erythema toxicum, neonatal urticaria). These lesions are sometimes confused with the uncommon but potentially serious staphylococcal sepsis (pemphigus). Where there is doubt the contents of a vesicle should be smeared on a microscope slide and a Gram stain performed. Eosinophils will be seen in cases of neonatal urticaria and Gram-positive cocci in pemphigus. When micro-organisms are seen, a culture should be collected and the infant started on antibiotics. Otherwise, it is important to check that the baby is apyrexial, feeding well, and that there are no signs of local infection. In these cases, simple reassurance is indicated.

Causes of vesicular rashes

chickenpox;
dermatitis herpetiformis;
hand, foot, and mouth disease;
herpes simplex and eczema herpeticum;
herpes zoster;
impetigo;
insect bites;
molluscum contagiosum.

(Note: drug eruptions and allergic reactions can, but rarely do, cause vesicular rashes.)

The important diagnostic features of conditions associated with rashes are tabulated in Table 2 and described below where the condition is not covered in the Diseases section.

Dermatitis herpetiformis

There is no prodromal illness or general malaise but symmetrical erythematous itchy vesicles appear gradually over the trunk,

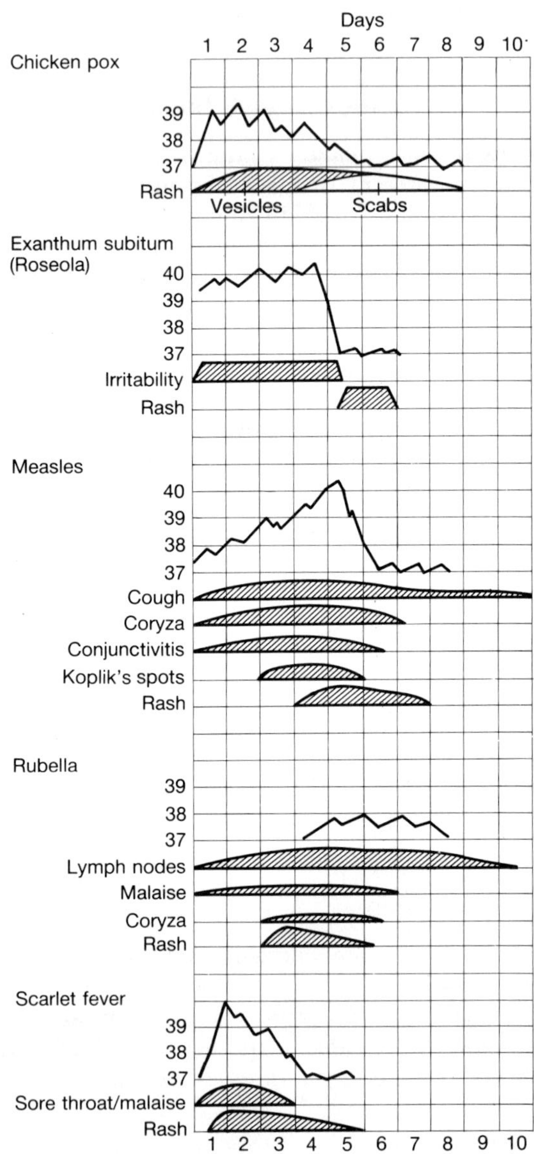

Fig. 2 Diagnostic clinical features of five commoner infections causing a rash.

Table 2 Diagnostic features of common rashes

	Prodrome	Fever	General malaise	Distribution of rash	Itchy	Special features
Vesicular rashes						
Chickenpox	None or short coryzal	Mild	Mild	Mostly trunk	Yes	Contact with other sufferers is common; crops
Dermatitis herpetiformis	Nil	Nil	Nil	Trunk	Yes	Sporadic cases eventually leave depigmentation
Eczema herpeticum	Nil	Moderate	Moderate	In areas of eczema	Yes	May be seriously ill
Hand, foot, and mouth	Nil	Minimal	Minimal	Palm, soles, and inside mouth	No	Often in minor epidemics
H. simplex (gingivostomatitis)	Nil	Mild	Moderate	Mouth and lips	Yes	Frequent history of contact with cold sores
Impetigo	Nil	Nil	Nil	Face and hands	Yes	Vesicles often replaced by yellow eruptions
Insect bites	Nil	Nil	Rare	Variable	Yes	Usually isolated lesions

Table 2 Diagnostic features of common rashes (*contd*)

	Prodrome	Fever	General malaise	Distribution of rash	Itchy	Special features
Molluscum contagiosum	Nil	Nil	Nil	Variable	No	Characteristic pearly vesicles with central dimple
Maculopapular and punctiform rashes						
Enteroviral infections	Short	Very mild	Mild	General	No	
Erythema infectiosum (Fifth disease, slapped cheeks syndrome)	Uncommon mild fever and respiratory symptoms	Mild if any	Minimal	Face 'slapped cheeks' and limbs	No	—
Exanthem subitum (roseola infantum, sixth disease)	High fever and irritability	High	Substantial	Trunk then face	No	The child improves dramatically when rash appears on 4th or 5th day

Glandular fever	Malaise, mild fever, and sore throat	Moderate	Common	General	No	Exudate in throat especially marked
Measles	Rising fever, cough, conjunctivitis	High	Substantial	Around ears then face, then trunk; confluent	No	Koplik's spots in mouth before rash on 4th day of illness
Meningococcal disease	None or short with coryza or fever	Variable	Profound	Variable	No	Petechial rash may be preceded by maculopapular rash
Kawasaki disease (Mucocutaneous lymph node syndrome)	Mild fever, malaise, sore throat	Mild	Mild to moderate	General	No	Palms and soles, lips and conjunctivae affected
Pityriasis rosea	Nil	Nil	Nil	Trunk	Initially	Usually older children; herald patch at onset
Rubella	Short, mild fever and malaise	Mild	Mild or nil	Face then trunk and limbs	No	Posterior occipital lymphadenopathy
Scarlet fever	Fever and sore throat	Yes	Moderate	Face then rapidly generalized	No	Rash blanches on pressure; strawberry tongue and peri-oral pallor

eventually resolving leaving dark pigmentation (or depigmentation on Asian or black skin).

Eczema herpeticum

The child has a history of eczema, sometimes of cold sores, is acutely unwell with fever and vesicular lesions in the eczematous areas.

Insect bites

Generally painful or itchy with an erythematous base but rarely with systemic disturbance.

Causes of maculopapular and punctiform rashes

enteroviral infections,
erythema infectiosum (fifth disease),
exanthem subitum (roseola infantum),
infectious mononucleosis,
measles,
meningococcal disease,
Kawasaki disease (mucocutaneous lymph node syndrome)
pityriasis rosea,
rubella,
scarlet fever.

(Note also: drug eruptions, malaria, sunburn, and contact allergies can cause maculopapular or punctiform rashes.)

The important diagnostic features are tabulated in Table 2 and described below where the condition is not covered in the Diseases section. See also Fig. 2, p. 14.

Enteroviral infections

A number of these viruses (coxsackie, echoviruses) produce a very mild fever and malaise which may precede, but more often coincide with the rash which is discrete (i.e. the macules do not run into one another), non-itchy and general in distribution.

Exanthem subitum (roseola infantum)

A disease showing a continuous high fever (up to 40°C) and irritability, which both subside with the appearance of a discrete maculopapular rash at 4–5 days. This is initially on the trunk and then spreads to the face and limbs. (See p. 102 and Fig. 2.)

Pityriasis rosea

This occurs in older (school-age) children. Initially a patch appears on the trunk looking like ringworm (the herald patch). Later there are more generalized red papules which merge to form an oval plaque which is initially itchy. This condition is not infectious to others.

Causes of haemorrhagic rashes

The rapid onset of a haemorrhagic rash suggests either meningococcal infection or a clotting disorder (e.g. idiopathic thrombocytopaenic purpura (ITP) or leukaemia). Urgent referral is necessary.

Other rashes

Scabies

This produces an itchy rash sometimes with papules and vesicles, most common around fingers, wrists and elbows. Linear burrows may be seen but are frequently hidden by the frantic scratching. Other family members are often affected. (See also p. 262.)

Itchy rashes

Itchiness and scratching are characteristic of the following:

chickenpox;
eczema;
hand, foot, and mouth disease;
herpes simplex;
impetigo;
insect bites.

The child with a fever

This section deals with cases in which the major, perhaps the only, presenting feature is a fever. Acute pyrexia will be considered first followed by persistent fever (pyrexia of unknown origin—PUO).

Acute fever

The commonest causes are (in approximately diminishing frequency): acute viral illness (various types); otitis media; tonsillitis; pneumonia; gastroenteritis; urinary-tract infection; bacteraemia; infectious hepatitis; meningitis; malaria; non-infectious conditions, e.g. connective tissue disorders.

A careful history has to be taken with emphasis on recent general health, other symptoms, contact with infections, travel abroad, and, in particular, present medication. A thorough examination must be performed to identify the more common infections. This will include ears, conjunctivae, throat, neck (for stiffness), chest, lymph nodes, and abdomen. (Palpation of a spleen may reveal that the 'tonsillitis' is in reality part of glandular fever.) The child must be undressed completely so that any rash may be observed.

If the child is only moderately unwell with signs of a viral infection (lymphadenopathy, injected conjunctivae, inflamed fauces, and rash) home care with symptomatic treatment can be given. Red eyes and ear-drums may arise from persistent crying rather than infection. Otitis media may be hard to diagnose because of difficulty in viewing the tympanic membranes. Where this is suspected but not confirmed the child should be re-examined later.

When no diagnosis can be made, but the child is obviously unwell, the more serious causes must be excluded by further examination (bones, joints, and soft tissues). A specific diagnosis may be particularly difficult to make in very young children (see p. 4) or if an antibiotic has already been given which could mask a serious infection. In these circumstances, referral to hospital is recommended. Where there is no obvious focus of infection in infancy or childhood, urinary-tract infection should be considered and a urine specimen collected (see p. 22). It may be necessary to review the child in a few hours.

If a decision is made to treat a baby or child at home, the family need instructions in how to manage a fever, the signs of deterioration, and what actions to take. These are best written down; some practitioners supply standard cards (as described on p. 4).

Persistent fever—PUO (pyrexia of unknown origin)

Technically this is defined as a temperature (over 38.5°C) lasting for more than 14 days without a diagnosis. However, any child with a fever for more than five days with no obvious cause requires referral to hospital. Infectious aetiologies remain the commonest causes of PUO; but fever may be a component of other illnesses.

Again, history and examination should be scrupulous. Investigations will depend on the clinical findings but must include urine microscopy and culture, full blood count and film, blood cultures, and, if the child has been to a malarious country, even if prophylaxis was given, a thick blood film.

Causes of persistent fever

Infective causes

Abscesses (dental, osteomyelitis, peritonsillar, appendix); bacteraemia; septic arthritis; endocarditis; infective hepatitis; glandular fever (infectious mononucleosis); Kawasaki disease (mucocutaneous lymph node syndrome); sinusitis; tuberculosis; typhoid fever; urinary-tract infection; listeriosis; brucellosis; malaria; relapsing fever.

Non-infective causes

Uncommon causes

Malignancy: leukaemia, lymphomas; gastrointestinal: ulcerative colitis, Crohn's disease; connective tissue disorders: systemic juvenile rheumatoid arthritis (Still's disease); antibiotic induced.

Rare causes

Malignancy: sarcoma, histiocytosis; connective tissue disorders: systemic lupus erythematosus (SLE), Behcet's syndrome, ectodermal dysplasia; factitious: Munchhausen by proxy syndrome; neurodegenerative disorders.

The child with urinary-tract infection

The diagnosis of urinary-tract infection (UTI) should be considered in any infant or child with fever, especially with rigors or vomiting. Dysuria, while a common symptom in the older child, cannot be declared under the age of two, and frequency is unlikely to be noted in the normally incontinent infant. Infection should be considered in the presence of nocturnal enuresis or when an established toiletting pattern breaks down.

Diagnosis is important, particularly under the age of five, because untreated infection in the presence of ureteric reflux may lead to renal scarring which, when severe, may progress to end-stage renal failure in later years. Early treatment should reduce the likelihood of renal damage.

Because it is so important to exclude UTI in a child with fever, antibiotics should not be given unless there is an obvious cause of infection (e.g. tonsillitis, pneumonia). The diagnosis of a suspected first UTI must be confirmed by microscopy and culture (testing for protein alone is unacceptable). If a urine specimen is not collected and sent to the laboratory for culture an important congenital renal abnormality may be missed. Furthermore, a paediatrician may subsequently be uncertain as to whether or not the child has had a urinary-tract infection and may feel obliged to arrange what can be unnecessary investigation. However, it is normal practice for paediatricians to arrange radiological investigations in all children under the age of one year following a single urinary-tract infection, and to investigate after either one or two infections in children up to the age of six.

During infancy the satisfactory collection of urine is a fine art. Clean catch specimens are probably best but require time, patience, and an appropriate receptacle (sterile jar) to hand. Urine specimens are frequently collected in adhesive sterile, disposable bags applied to the skin around the perineum. The perineum should be washed with water before the bag is applied. This is best done in a warm room with the bag exposed and the infant held upright so that as soon as urine is passed the bag can be removed and urine drained from a freshly cut hole into a sterile container. False negatives are uncommon using this technique but a high proportion of false positives will occur if the bag is left on too long, allowing contamination with bacteria from the perineal skin. In the toilet-trained child, specimens can be collected successfully by putting a sterile gallipot in a clean potty, and in older children an MSU can be taken.

Specimens should be sent to the laboratory immediately after collection. Failing this, they can be kept in a refrigerator (at 4°C) and sent the next day. When only a culture result is required a dipslide can be used: a plastic paddle coated with agar is dipped into the urine and then sent to the laboratory.

Urinary-tract infection can be diagnosed when a single bacterial strain is cultured with a count of 10^5 organisms/ml, or more. Most infections are associated with pyuria, that is more than 50 leucocytes (white blood cells) on microscopy. When this is the first occasion that infection is suspected in a young child, and the specimen has been collected into a bag, another sample should be obtained to confirm infection before antibiotics are given. This should be done by suprapubic aspiration in hospital, or clean catch. The specimen should be collected quickly, particularly in infancy when urinary infection can progress to septicaemia over a short period. Indeed, in a sick infant with suspected urinary-tract infection there is no place for a bag urine collection and a suprapubic aspiration of urine should be performed. In an older child with pyelonephritis (dysuria, fever, loin tenderness) there is less need for a second sample. A second sample should also be taken if there is a positive culture, but normal urine microscopy.

Most urinary-tract infections in children are caused by Gram-negative bowel commensals, especially *Escherichia coli*. When antibiotics need to be given before the culture results are available, trimethoprin or co-trimoxazole (sulphamethoxazole and trimethoprin) are the drugs of choice. Other antibiotics may be required once the results of sensitivity testing are available (amoxycillin, cephradine and nitrofurantoin). Antibiotic treatment should continue for five days.

Prophylactic antibiotic treatment may be given to some infants and young children thought to be at risk of further infection, particularly where there are known to be congenital renal abnormalities or where ureteric reflux has been demonstrated by investigation. A urine culture should be performed 3–5 days after treatment has been discontinued, or during prophylactic treatment. Care should be taken with the interpretation of urine results in children on antibiotics; pyuria alone may be the only indication that infection is still present. Children with a first infection, particularly under the age of five, should be referred to a paediatrician who will then decide on further investigations; referral should be urgent in children under the age of one year, who will need a suprapubic aspiration or clean-catch urine collection as soon as a urinary infection is thought to be present.

The parents of children with UTIs should be advised to encourage plentiful fluids during episodes of infection. Careful attention should be paid to toilet hygiene, and bubble baths, which may promote irritation and lead to further infection, should be discouraged, particularly for girls.

The child with vomiting and diarrhoea

Vomiting

The commonest cause of vomiting is gastrointestinal infection and is often associated with diarrhoea. Vomiting may be a symptom of other childhood conditions which may need urgent investigation and treatment, such as meningitis and urinary-tract infection.

Causes other than gastroenteritis to be considered are listed below.

Vomiting of central origin

Meningitis, encephalitis, intracranial-space-occupying lesion, migraine, Reye's syndrome.

Vomiting from gastrointestinal disease

(1) In the newborn: intestinal obstruction from small-bowel atresia, meconium ileus, Hirschsprung's disease, malrotation, volvulus;
(2) in infancy: pyloric stenosis, intussusception, appendicitis, oesophageal hiatus hernia;
(3) in childhood: appendicitis, malrotation, oesophageal stricture.

Metabolic causes

Congenital adrenal hyperplasia, Addison's disease, diabetic ketoacidosis, uraemia in renal failure.

Other causes

Drugs and toxins, periodic syndrome, pregnancy in adolescent girls, as part of systemic infections, tonsillitis, otitis media, urinary-tract infection, measles, hepatitis.

The causes listed above should be considered and eliminated by careful history and examination before a diagnosis of gastroenteritis is made. For instance, a vomiting child with fever and neck stiffness is likely to have meningitis, fever with rigors, urinary tract infection, and where the vomiting is bile stained intestinal obstruction is likely.

When the child appears unwell and there is no clear cause referral to hospital may be indicated. This is the case for persistent vomiting, particularly in infancy, which may lead quickly to electrolyte imbalance. **There is no place for anti-emetic drugs in the vomiting child.**

Diarrhoea

In early infancy babies (especially if breast fed) may have frequent soft even watery stools. Older children can have 'toddler diarrhoea' (persistent loose stools containing undigested food in a well child growing normally).

Diarrhoea is rarely due to disease beyond the gastro-intestinal tract. Although most causes of acute change in bowel habit are due to local infections the causes listed below need to be considered particularly where the diarrhoea is prolonged. A useful sign is that with the exception of malabsorptive conditions (eg cystic fibrosis) foul-smelling stools generally indicate infection.

Conditions where diarrhoea can be a presenting feature

(1) During infancy: drugs (especially antibiotics), lactose or cows' milk protein intolerance, urinary-tract infection, coeliac disease, cystic fibrosis, appendicitis;
(2) during childhood: drugs, laxatives; appendicitis; ulcerative colitis; Crohn's disease; haemolytic uraemic syndrome; mucocutaneous lymph node syndrome (Kawasaki disease).

For both vomiting and/or diarrhoea, once a diagnosis of gastroenteritis has been made, further management should proceed as described on p. 56.

The child with bacterial meningitis

Introduction

Despite advances in treatment for this condition it remains the most important bacterial cause of mortality and morbidity in children in this country.

Epidemiology

This is predominantly a disease of neonates and very young children. In the post-natal period the incidence is 65/100 000 in the under 1–11 month age group and 16/100 000 in the 1–4 year age group. The most common causative organisms at various ages are shown in Table 3.

Clinical features

The onset of symptoms may be relatively insidious or there may be rapid progression with coma and prostration. Meningitis may present with fever, vomiting, lethargy, and, in the younger child, convulsions. In the older child headache, vomiting, and anorexia are common presenting symptoms. However, with slower onset illness, the symptoms and signs are often non-specific, especially in very young children. Doctors dealing with young children with acute febrile illnesses should have a high index of suspicion and a low threshold for performing a lumbar puncture. Whereas in the older child neck stiffness is the characteristic sign, this may not be present in the child under 18 months. The classical purpuric rash of meningococcal sepsis occurs in about half to two-thirds of cases of meningitis caused by this organism. However, such a rash may occasionally be caused by the other meningitic pathogens. A non-specific maculopapular rash may also occur in meningococcal disease. Arthritis may complicate Haemophilus and Meningococcal meningitis and in the latter is often multifocal.

Table 3 Common causative organisms of bacterial meningitis

Age	Common cause	Empirical antibiotic treatment
0–1 month	Group B *Streptoccocus* *Escherichia coli* (usually K1 serotype) *Listeria monocytogenes*	Ampicillin and Gentamicin or Cefotaxime and Ampicillin
1–3 months	*Neisseria meningitidis* *Haemophilus influenzae* type B (Hib) *Streptoccocus pneumoniae* Group B *Steptoccocus* *Escherichia coli* *Listeria monocytogenes*	Cefotaxime and Ampicillin
3 months–5 years	*Neisseria meningitidis* *Haemophilus influenzae* type B (Hib) *Streptoccocus pneumoniae*	Ampicillin/ Penicillin and Chloramphenicol or Cefotaxime
6 years or more	*Neisseria meningitidis* *Streptococcus pneumoniae*	

See appendix for dosages.

Natural history

Outside the neonatal period, the causative organisms are spread by respiratory secretions and droplet transmission. Usually the bacteria first colonize the nasopharynx and from there invade via the blood to the meninges. Asymptomatic nasopharyngeal carriers of these organisms are not uncommon in the population. Pneumococcal meningitis may be associated with chronic middle ear sepsis, may follow skull fractures, or may complicate congenital defects in the coverings of the central nervous system.

Diagnosis

Lumbar puncture with cerebrospinal fluid examination provides the basis for diagnosis. A gram stain and cell count should be performed. In cases of bacterial meningitis, more than 50 WBC cu/mm is usual, although more than 20 is abnormal. Polymorphonuclear leucocyte should predominate: mononuclear cells are seen in tuberculous and viral meningitis, and partially treated cases of bacterial infection. Tuberculous and viral cases should be differentiated by history, and clinical signs. In tuberculous infection as with bacterial meningitis CSF glucose is low, and protein elevated. In meningococcal sepsis gram stain and/or culture of material obtained from skin lesions may be used to confirm the diagnosis. Antigen detection tests such as the latex agglutination test may detect bacterial products in CSF, blood, or urine and enable identification of the causative organism to be made when cultures are negative. These may be particularly useful if prior antibiotic therapy was given or if lumbar puncture is contraindicated because of raised intracranial pressure.

Management

Children with suspected meningococcal sepsis should be given parenteral benzyl penicillin or ampicillin prior to transfer to hospital. In hospital, blood culture and lumbar puncture should be performed without delay and intravenous antibiotics commenced. It is acceptable to give these before lumbar puncture when there are clinical signs of meningococcal infection. The fundi should be examined for evidence of papilloedema before a lumbar puncture is performed. In the unconscious child, intracranial pressure may be high, even in the absence of papilloedema, and a lumbar puncture may increase the risk of coning. In these cases lumbar puncture should be avoided. Nevertheless, treatment of presumed meningitis without a bacteriological diagnosis is unsatisfactory, and because other serious illness may have similar signs, management of this condition without a lumbar puncture should be the exception rather than the rule. Outside the neonatal period penicillin or ampicillin and chloramphenicol or cefotaxime is recommended (see Table 1 and appendix). Because of the emergence of chloramphenicol- and ampicillin-resistant strains of *H. influenzae*, some clinicians are using cefotaxime (see Appendix 2). When a penicillin chloramphenicol combination is used it is recommended that both antibiotics are given together until the results of culture are obtained, rather than relying on a gram stain alone. Clearly this advice does not apply when additional information is provided by a positive latex agglutination test. Complications of meningitis include cerebral oedema, and inappropriate antidiuretic hormone secretion. Fluids should be restricted during the early stage of infection.

Chemoprophylaxis for close contacts and the index case using rifampicin to eliminate nasopharyngeal carriage is used following infections with meningococcus and *Haemophilus influenzae* type b (see p. 90 and p. 67).

Long-term complications include sensorineural deafness (approximately 5–10 per cent of cases) as well as motor and intellectual impairment. Children should be followed up, and hearing tests performed.

The child with bone and joint infection

Acute osteomyelitis, an infection of the bone, usually arises by haematogenous spread of bacteria and most commonly arises in the metaphyseal region of one of the larger bones. It may spread to involve the adjacent joint, giving rise to an accompanying pyogenic arthritis. Rarely it may be multifocal. About 10 per cent of cases arise by direct extension from an adjacent infected focus or from a penetrating injury.

Acute pyogenic arthritis may occur as an extension of osteomyelitis, or may arise by haematogenous spread without any overt signs of bony involvement. Most cases are monarticular (usually hip, knee, ankle, or elbow) but in about 10 per cent of cases several joints are affected.

Aetiology

The majority (approximately 80 per cent) of acute bone and joint infections are caused by *Staphylococcus aureus*. The primary focus of staphylococcal infection leading to bacteraemia is usually not evident. In the 3 months to 5 years age group *Haemophilus influenzae* type B (Hib) is also an important cause of septic arthritis (and to a lesser extent osteomyelitis). Gram-negative enteric bacilli, salmonella species, Group A haemolytic streptococcus and *Streptococcus pneumoniae* are other important causes. Gram-negative enteric bacilli are more likely to be the cause in immunocompromised individuals such as neonates, those with immune deficiency, or sickle-cell diseases. Group B *Streptococcus* is another important neonatal cause. *Neisseria gonorrhoea* may cause pyogenic arthritis, particularly when perinatally acquired.

Clinical features

In acute cases there is usually a short history (< 24 hours), the child is ill-looking and feverish. There is a refusal to move the affected limb or to bear weight on an affected leg. In osteomyelitis there is usually swelling overlying the bone and tenderness. In pyogenic arthritis the affected joint may be hot, swollen, and tender.

Diagnosis and management

In most acute cases the diagnosis can be made clinically. Investigations will show a raised white cell count, sedimentation rate, and C reactive protein. (The last two are useful in monitoring response to treatment.) Radiographs initially show no bony changes but may show soft tissue swelling and joint effusions. If there is doubt an isotope bone scan will confirm an inflammatory process in joint or bone. Blood cultures (multiple if possible) should be taken, and are positive in approximately 40 per cent of cases of pyogenic arthritis and 60 per cent of acute osteomyelitis. Antigen detection tests to *H. influenzae* and antigen in urine or joint fluid may help to identify the cause. Tests for anti-staphylococcal antibody are generally disappointing in children.

The mainstay of treatment is appropriate antibiotic therapy with or without surgical intervention. In pyogenic arthritis, drainage of the joint should always be performed and is both therapeutically and diagnostically useful. Needle aspiration is an important diagnostic test. In acute osteomyelitis with a short history, no bony changes on radiographs, and no underlying disease, it is reasonable to treat empirically with antibiotics, with surgical exploration reserved for cases which fail to respond clinically or develop complications.

The differential diagnosis of osteomyelitis or septic arthritis may include non-pyogenic infections (eg tuberculosis or virus), juvenile rheumatoid arthritis, and leukaemia. If the child has an underlying disorder, the infecting organism may be unusual. Therefore in these cases primary surgical exploration is usually indicated.

Initial antibiotic treatment should be given intravenously in high dosage. Empirical treatment before culture results are available should be given with flucloxacillin, fucidin, and ampicillin (or cefotaxime to cover β lactamase producing strains of *H. influenzae*.

When culture results are available, antibiotics can be modified—the combination of flucloxacillin and fucidin provides good anti-staphylococcal treatment while ampicillin is used for Streptococcal and non β lactamase producing Haemophilus infections.

Other antibiotics which may be useful are clindamycin or 2nd Generation cephalosporins. In salmonella osteomyelitis ampicillin, cotrimoxazole or ciprofloxacin may be used, depending on the sensitivity of the organism. Intravenous antibiotic therapy should be continued for a minimum of three days or until the fever has been settled for 48 hours, whichever is the longer. Thereafter oral antibiotic therapy is continued for 3–4 weeks for septic arthritis or 4–6 weeks in osteomyelitis. Measurement of serum bactericidal levels may be useful in ensuring adequate oral therapy, especially when there is an unusual causal organism or there is evidence of persisting inflammation (eg persisting high ESR or CRP). In chronic osteomyelitis very prolonged antibiotic treatment as well as surgery is required.

The child with sexually transmitted disease

Microbiological tests and their use in providing possible evidence of sexual abuse

Evidence for sexually transmitted diseases may be sought in children suffering from anal, penile, and vaginal warts, vaginal or urethral discharges, or when there is a history of contact with an individual with a known or possible genital infection. The recommended investigations are summarized in Table 4. Where genital warts are seen, it is recommended that they are removed (under general anaesthesia in the young child) and sent for typing. Rapid diagnostic tests for *Chlamydia trachomatis*, such as the enzyme-linked immunosorbent assay (ELISA) and immunofluorescence, may be unreliable and the diagnosis should be confirmed by cell culture. Results of *Neisseria gonorrhoeae* culture may need to be confirmed by a reference laboratory.

Gonorrhoea, perianal warts, and *Chlamydia* infections outside the immediate newborn period are strongly suggestive of sexual contact. If child sexual abuse is suspected, then it is important that the specimens are handled to meet the requirements for collecting forensic evidence, that is, the person who takes the specimen and all subsequent people who handle it should sign the label to ensure continuity of evidence. If child sexual abuse is suspected, it would be appropriate for the child to be assessed by a doctor with relevant experience. It is currently recommended that a full examination in a paediatric setting is performed by a paediatrician and an experienced police surgeon.

For a more detailed discussion of *N. gonorrhoeae* infection see p. 64; for *C. trachomatis* see p. 46; and herpes simplex virus p. 75.

Table 4 Investigations to be performed for diagnosis of sexually transmitted agents in childhood; detection of one or more of these agents from the genital tract in infancy or childhood indicates probable sexual abuse

Organism/lesion	Site of specimen	Transport to laboratory on	Recommended isolation/confirmation	Comments
Neisseria gonorrhoeae	vagina penile urethra anus fauces	charcoal swab	culture on agar	
Chlamydia trachomatis	vagina penile urethra anus (remove pus before specimen collected)	swab in Chlamydia transport medium and smear on microscope slide	cell culture immunofluorescence	Always confirm with culture if rapid diagnostic test is positive
Trichomonas vaginalis	vagina	charcoal swab or trichomonas culture medium	microscopy culture	
Herpes simplex virus (HSV)/genital herpes	vagina penile urethra anus	swab in viral transport medium	tissue culture electron microscopy	Reactivation of lesions occurs
Human papilloma virus (HPV), condyloma acuminata (wart)	anus vagina penis	rapid transit and freeze at -70°C (biopsy specimen)	histology electron microscopy	DNA analysis may be available for identification of genital HPV strains

Congenital infections

Management of important infections during pregnancy and the neonatal period

Table 5

Organism/ disease	Management in pregnancy	Management of newborn
Chlamydia trachomatis	Treat parents with erythromycin	Tetracycline to eyes, oral erythromycin
Cytomegalovirus (CMV)	Rarely diagnosed; symptoms mild.	Symptomatic
Enterovirus	No action if in early pregnancy	Isolate newborn from other infants where intra-partum infection
Hepatitis B	—	Hepatitis B immune globulin and vaccine where mother HBeAg positive and anti-HBe negative (see p. 166); immunize infants of all HBsAg mothers; barrier nurse (see Glossary) where mother e antigen positive
Herpes simplex virus (HSV) (genital)	Greatest risk in 1° infection; Caesarean section where lesions present	Acyclovir in definite or suspected infection; isolate
Human immuno-deficiency virus (HIV) AIDS/ARC	Consider termination of pregnancy because of high risk of congenital infection	Isolation unnecessary; extreme care with blood (see p. 42)

Organism/ disease	Management in pregnancy	Management of newborn
Listeria monocytogenes Listeriosis	Ampicillin 4–6 g/day in acute infection	Ampicillin plus gentamicin
Measles	No action required	—(Extremely rare)
Mumps	No action required	—(Extremely rare)
Mycobacterium tuberculosis/ Tuberculosis (TB)	Positive tuberculin test and positive CXR needs treatment	Isolate infant from mother with active TB until she is non-contagious and give isoniazid (INAH) and INAH-resistant BCG; give INAH and rifampicin to infant with TB
Neisseria gonorrhoea/ gonorrhoea	Ampicillin or benzyl penicillin or cefuroxime iv	Single dose of benzyl penicillin where untreated maternal infection and asymptomatic infant; treat neonatal infection with benzyl penicillin iv for seven days
Rubella*	Counsel for possible termination following infection before 18 weeks' gestation	Symptomatic; early hearing tests
Streptococcus agalactiae Group B	Ampicillin 2 g every 4 h where amnionitis and when colonized	Benzyl penicillin intravenously
Toxoplasma gondii/ toxoplasmosis	Rarely diagnosed (see p. 119) Spiramycin pyramethamine and sulpha diazine	Courses of pyrimethamine, sulphadiazine, folinic acid, and spiramycin (see p. 121)

Organism/ disease	Management in pregnancy	Management of newborn
Treponema pallidum/ Syphilis	Treat with benzyl penicillin, (a) clinical disease +/−pos VDRL (venereal disease research laboratory) (b) and pos VDRL with pos FTA-ABS (fluorescent treponemal antibody)	
Varicella/ chickenpox	Zoster immuno-globulin (ZIG) can be given to pregnant varicella contacts when no previous history and seronegative. Termination of pregnancy not indicated	ZIG essential when maternal infection 7 days before to 7 days after delivery; PHLS will supply ZIG for infants when maternal infection up to 1 month after birth; give acyclovir alone for neonatal infection; observe for 10 days after onset of rash in mother. ZIG indicated for infant preterm less than 28 weeks' gestation.

Breast feeding should be encouraged for infants with congenital infection. Although HIV has been isolated from breast milk there is no evidence that infection has been transmitted to the newborn, except where infection has been acquired postnatally. In the UK, where infants cows' milk formulae are available, artificial feeding may be preferred.

* To diagnose acute maternal rubella infection provide paired sera to demonstrate rise in rubella antibody, the first taken within 2–3 days of onset of the rash and the second from 8–9 days after the onset; alternatively provide a single sample from seven days to six weeks after the onset for estimation of rubella-specific IgM. Provide the laboratory with a full clinical history. All suspected cases of congenital rubella syndrome must be notified to the National Congenital Rubella Surveillance Scheme (see p. 106).

Diseases

AIDS (Acquired immunodeficiency syndrome)/HIV infection

Organism

The human immunodeficiency virus (HIV).

Epidemiology

AIDS is not a notifiable disease and figures are based on laboratory reports of HIV-positive results and voluntary clinical case reporting to the British Paediatric Surveillance Unit (BPSU), the Communicable Disease Surveillance Centre (CDSC), or the Communicable Disease Unit (Scotland). Paediatricians and other doctors managing HIV-positive children and paediatric AIDS cases should ensure that they are reported to the relevant body.

By the end of December 1989 there had been 359 laboratory reports in the UK of children (under age 15) having blood positive for antibody to HIV (see Table 6). In addition, 43 cases of childhood AIDS had been reported (Table 7).

The two main groups of children infected in the UK were cases where transmission was from mother to child (vertical transmission) and others infected by transfusion of blood products or blood itself. In addition, there are a small number of paediatric AIDS cases where transmission occurred outside the UK and others where information is insufficient to determine the route of infection.

The most important source of infection in a child is from its mother. Women at highest risk of HIV infection are:

- drug abusers who have injected themselves since 1977;
- sexual partners of such drug abusers;
- sexual partners of bisexual men;
- women who had a transfusion or sex with men living in Africa south of the countries bordering on the Mediterranean in countries where AIDS is endemic;
- prostitutes;
- sexual partners of haemophiliacs.

Table 6 Paediatric HIV-antibody positive reports to December 1989

HIV-1 Antibody positive reports Exposure category	< 1y	1–4y	5–9y	10–14y	Total
Parent HIV infected/at risk	120	34	1	—	155
Blood/components recipient					
abroad	—	1	2	1	4
UK	—	1	1	2	4
undetermined	—	1	1	2	4
Haemophiliac	—	11	66	101	178
Other/undetermined	3	5	1	5	14
Total	123	53	72	111	359

The majority of women in the above risk groups will not be infected. Also, women may not realize that they are within the risk groups, and HIV infection occurs in women outside these groups. The highest risk is amongst women associated with injected drug abuse, amongst whom HIV-infection prevalence varies geographically. There is a particularly high rate, and hence a concentration of infected children, in Lothian (Scotland).

Transmission

Vertical transmission is the commonest source of new cases of HIV infection. Prenatal transmission occurs and transmission at birth through exposure to maternal blood seems likely. The role of breast feeding is under study. Kissing, close proximity, and other casual contacts do **NOT** lead to infection. With the exclusion of high-risk donors, the screening of donated blood for antibody as well as heat treatment of some blood products (Factor VIII), the risk of HIV infection following transfusion is very low. Infection can be transmitted following transfusion of infected blood before sero conversion of the donor has occurred.

Table 7 Paediatric AIDS cases to December 1989

AIDS cases Exposure category	Residents < 1y	 1–4y	 5–9y	 10–14y	Visitors 14y or less	Total
Parent HIV infected/at risk	9	10	1	—	4	24
Blood/components recipient						
abroad		1	1	—	2	4
UK		1	—	—	—	1
Haemophiliac		—	6	7	1	14
TOTAL	9	12	8	7	7	43

Figures, supplied by CDSC, include those for Scotland and Northern Ireland (note: more recent information than provided by BSPU).

Incubation period

(From exposure to antibody production) in adults infected by transfusion is approximately six weeks (median period); much longer periods have been reported in some children.

Infectivity

Apart from through the transfusion and vertical routes, infectivity is very low, considerably less than for hepatitis B. It is important for HIV-positive children to be treated as other children, and it must be appreciated that properly applied normal standards of infection control will prevent spread of the disease in the hospital and community. The Multicentre European Study has found a vertical transmission rate of approximately 25 per cent, with indications that women with symptomatic HIV infection are more likely to have infected babies.

Natural history

There is a spectrum of HIV infection from entirely asymptomatic cases through to AIDS itself. The majority of children infected through transfusion have developed some abnormality, and the median time from transfusion to AIDS is estimated to be two years. The manifestations of HIV infection in children are variable and considerably different from adults. Children who become symptomatic may present with any one or a combination of the following: recurrent bacterial infections, failure to thrive, persistent and recurrent severe oral candida (thrush), persistent or recurrent diarrhoea, generalized lymphadenopathy, enlarged liver and spleen (hepatosplenomegaly), progressive encephalopathy, or loss of developmental milestones.

Diagnosis

Because of the persistence of maternal antibody it is particularly difficult to diagnose HIV infection in children under 15 months. Virus isolation or antigen detection can help but is usually only available in specialist centres. Children found to be HIV positive under 15 months but who are asymptomatic, have no immunological abnormalities, and have not had isolation of virus or antigen detection, are referred to as having 'indeterminate' status. Conventional antibody testing is usually by an ELISA but a positive result must then be confirmed by a second independent test (using either another type of ELISA or a Western blot test). For these and other reasons, diagnosis of both HIV positivity and paediatric AIDS is complicated and specialist advice must be sought.

See p. 217 for immunization of HIV-positive children.

Childhood HIV infection has only been recognized in the past few years and knowledge about it is rapidly accumulating. Hence, policy on management and care are changing and are not appropriate for detailed discussion in a book such as this. Readers are advised to consult the guidelines published by the Royal College of Obstetricians and Gynaecologists and the British Paediatric Association (Further reading, nos 18 and 19, p. 273). Recommendations include the following:

Childbirth

Gloves, gowns, masks, and goggles should be used by staff assisting in childbirth when a woman is known to be HIV positive, or is in a high risk group.

Staff with open wounds or eczema on the hands should cover the affected areas with waterproof plasters or gloves when caring for a high risk mother in childbirth, or her infant.

Paediatricians attending high risk deliveries should wear masks, disposable gowns, surgical gloves, and safety spectacles.

Only mechanical suction should be used. The infant should be washed free of blood and liquor after delivery.

Careful attention should be paid to disinfection of non-disposable apparatus (1 per cent sodium hypochlorite to be used).

The infant receiving intensive care

Extreme care should be used in practical procedures such as venesection and insertion of catheters into blood vessels. Staff should cover open wounds on their hands and when feasible gloves should be worn.

Breast feeding

It is suggested that HIV positive mothers in the UK should bottle feed their infants. However there is no evidence to suggest that breast feeding increases the risk of transmission of infection to the newborn, except in the very rare cases of postnatally acquired infection. This recommendation should not be adopted in developing countries, where women should be encouraged to breast feed.

Immunization

BCG should not be given to an HIV positive infant, or to an infant of an HIV positive mother.

Oral polio vaccine (OPV) can be given to an HIV positive infant. However, if another member of the family is immunocompromised killed polio vaccine (IPV) should be used.

Measles vaccine and the measles, mumps, rubella vaccine (MMR) should be administered to HIV positive infants.

Diphtheria, pertussis and tetanus vaccines are indicated.

Chickenpox (varicella) and Herpes zoster (shingles)

Organism

Herpes virus—varicella/zoster; a DNA virus.

Epidemiology

Chickenpox is highly infectious so that most children become infected and remain immune into adulthood. Infection in childhood is normally benign but may be severe in the immunosuppressed child, and in the newborn infant when infection develops in the mother close to the time of delivery.

Transmission

is by direct contact, droplet infection or recently soiled materials, e.g. handkerchiefs.

Incubation period

is from 14 to 21 days.

Period of infectivity

is from one day prior to eruption of the rash and then for six days after the rash appears.

Natural history of infection in childhood and pregnancy

Primary infection with the virus results in chickenpox. There may be a short (less than 24 hours) coryzal prodrome followed by fever and an itchy vesicular rash. Crops of vesicles, sparser on the limbs than trunk, appear over 3–5 days.

Complications are unusual but include thrombocytopenia and encephalitis. Aspirin given during this illness is thought to increase the risk of Reye's syndrome. Immunosuppressed children have continued cropping of lesions as well as encephalitis, pancreatitis, hepatitis, and pneumonia. Infection during early pregnancy may result in varicella embryopathy.

Reactivation of the virus which lies latent in a spinal nerve root may occur in both children and adults, and results in shingles or zoster, a painful rash where vesicles are grouped in a dermatome pattern (a dermatome is an area of skin served by a single spinal nerve).

Diagnosis

The diagnosis should be made on clinical features, but virus in vesicle fluid can be identified by electron microscopy or virus culture.

Management

Symptomatic treatment only is required in childhood **but aspirin should never be used as an antipyretic**. Children with chickenpox should not be admitted to hospital unless absolutely necessary because of the risk to immunosuppressed children. Infants and children with varicella should be barrier nursed.

The immunosuppressed child should be given zoster immune globulin (ZIG) if known to be varicella seronegative and in close contact with a case of chickenpox or shingles. If lesions appear, then oral acyclovir should be used; ZIG is of no value at this stage. Where pregnant women are exposed to varicella–zoster and they are susceptible then ZIG should be given. This will not prevent illness but reduce the severity of disease when given up to 10 days after contact.

Congenital varicella

This is rare and results in scarring of the skin, hypoplasia of bone and muscle normally in one limb, malformations of the central nervous system and eyes. Infection during pregnancy is not an indication for abortion.

Neonatal varicella—natural history and treatment

This is uncommon and babies are only at risk when the mother develops chickenpox between seven days before and seven days after delivery. It presents as a vesicular rash and there is a high mortality from varicella pneumonia. ZIG should be given to the newborn if the mother develops varicella during the risk period.

Acyclovir (intravenous or oral) is indicated following development of lesions in the newborn and is sometimes used in the mother and in her baby prophylactically where maternal infection occurs just before delivery. Infants exposed to Varicella delivered before 28 weeks' gestation should be given ZIG if still in hospital.

Chlamydia trachomatis

C. trachomatis **ophthalmia neonatorum is notifiable**

Organism

Chlamydia trachomatis. Some serotypes cause endemic trachoma and others sexually transmitted infections. This is a bacterial agent with an intra-cellular life cycle.

Epidemiology

This is the commonest cause of sexually transmitted infection in the UK. Infection is acquired during sexual intercourse or parturition. If the mother is infected, up to 50 per cent of infants develop conjunctivitis after delivery and almost half of untreated infants with conjunctivitis will develop pneumonia. *C. trachomatis* ophthalmia is more common than that due to the gonococcus and is notifiable. Identification in the genital tract of children implies sexual abuse.

Natural history

A purulent neonatal conjunctivitis may develop 5–14 days after birth and cannot be distinguished on clinical appearances from gonococcal or other infection. Inadequate treatment may result in recurrence and, rarely, in corneal scarring. Pneumonia may develop 4–6 weeks after birth and is associated with poor feeding, a cough, and tachypnoea. The chest X-ray shows hyper-inflation and generalized patchy shadowing. Pneumonia, although requiring treatment, is often self-limiting, but the outcome may be more serious in the preterm infant with coexistent chronic lung disease (bronchopulmonary dysplasia). Infection in the adolescent may lead to non-specific/non-gonococcal urethritis (NSU, NGU) and, in the female, salpingitis and possible infertility.

Diagnosis

A Gram stain on the exudate should be performed quickly in all cases of purulent conjunctivitis, to exclude gonococcal infection. Because *C. trachomatis* is an intra-cellular bacterium the specimen should include cells from the conjunctivae collected by firmly drawing a cotton-wool swab over the everted lower eyelid. Rapid diagnostic tests using monoclonal antibodies have been introduced and allow diagnosis of *C. trachomatis* from a smear on a microscope slide. An enzyme-linked immunosorbent assay is also available (ELISA). All these tests, but particularly the ELISA, may yield false positive results and for this reason the definitive tissue-culture test should be performed when there is a suspicion of sexually transmitted disease in children, following sexual abuse. The rapid diagnostic tests may be too insensitive to detect organisms in nasopharyngeal or tracheal aspirate for diagnosis of pneumonia, but are recommended for use in conjunctivitis.

Treatment

A topical eye preparation (e.g. tetracycline) can be used in combination with oral erythromycin in treatment of *Chlamydia ophthalmia*. Erythromycin must be given to reduce the risk of relapse of conjunctivitis when a topical preparation is discontinued, and to prevent development of pneumonia. Erythromycin is used for treatment of pneumonia (dose as above) and there is good evidence that it can be used alone in management of ophthalmia. Children with genital infections should be treated with erythromycin, and adolescents with tetracycline. Parents of infants with neonatal ophthalmia should be investigated and treated in a genito-urinary disease clinic.

Cholera

Notifiable disease

Organism

Widespread epidemic disease is associated only with *Vibrio cholerae* 0-group 1, a Gram-negative motile rod. Other groups may cause severe diarrhoea.

Epidemiology

Since 1961 cholera has spread from India and Southeast Asia to Africa, the Middle East, and even some parts of southern Europe.

Transmission

from an infected person is through contaminated water and food. Shellfish are important vehicles of transmission. With modern sanitation, widespread epidemics are less frequent but may follow natural disasters where there is contamination of food and water and a breakdown of hygiene and sanitation.

Incubation period

is 1–3 days with a range of a few hours to five days. The greater the dose of infecting organisms ingested the shorter the incubation period and the more severe the disease.

Period of infectivity

is variable, and a carrier state may last several months.

Natural history

Illness is characterized by the rapid onset of severe diarrhoea followed by vomiting. Profuse, frequent, and surprisingly painless bowel evacuations accelerate the severe dehydration, shock, and collapse that are the hallmarks of the disease.

Complications of delayed treatment are hypovolaemic shock, uncompensated metabolic acidosis, and renal failure, which have a high mortality. However, with improvements in treatment mortality has fallen and should be less than 5 per cent.

Diagnosis

In endemic areas, especially during epidemics, there is no difficulty in diagnosis but sporadic cases will require differentiation from other forms of severe diarrhoea. Diagnosis can be made by microscopic examination of the stool. Culture on bile-salt agar will produce characteristic colonies in 24 hours. The organism can be typed by agglutination with specific antisera. Specific antibody titres can also be measured.

Management

The most important aspect of treatment is the rapid restoration of plasma volume and electrolyte balance. Antibiotics are used for eradication of *Vibrio cholerae* from the gastro-intestinal tract. Co-trimoxazole should be given to children under 10 years of age, and tetracycline to older children (see p. 60 for dosage). The infected child needs to be barrier nursed during the acute phase, and special care taken with handling of stools (enteric precautions—see Glossary) until demonstrated to be non-infectious. Stools of close contacts should be cultured and carriers should be given antibiotics (treatment dose). Attempts must be made to identify the source of infection and appropriate control measures taken.

Cryptosporidiosis

Organism

Cryptosporidium is a coccidian protozoa.

Epidemiology

Cryptosporidiosis was considered until recently to be a disease only of the immunosuppressed. It is now recognized as an important cause of diarrhoea in normal children, accounting for 5 per cent of cases in 1–4 year-olds.

Transmission

Transmission is by ingestion of oocysts from infected hosts; these include farm animals, domestic pets (and other humans). Cases have been traced to unpasteurized cows' milk, contaminated mains water supplies, and outbreaks have been reported from children's nurseries, suggesting direct human-to-human transmission.

Incubation period

Not known.

Infectivity

While still excreting the cysts.

Natural history

Infection presents with watery diarrhoea, abdominal pain, vomiting, and fever. Although most children recover by the end of the second week of illness, in some, diarrhoea is more prolonged. Immunosuppressed children may develop debilitating illness, requiring interruption or modification of chemotherapy.

Diagnosis

This is by staining and microscopic examination of a faecal smear.

Treatment

Symptomatic in normal children. Spiramycin has been used with success in immunocompromised children. The British National Formulary preparation has an unpleasant taste, but a more palatable version is available by arrangement with the manufacturer.

Cytomegalovirus (CMV)

Organism

Cytomegalovirus (CMV). This is a DNA virus and is a member of the herpes group.

Epidemiology

Up to 50 per cent of individuals have had CMV infection (normally asymptomatic) by childbearing age in industrialized countries. Congenital CMV acquired transplacentally normally follows primary infection in the mother, although reactivation of maternal infection accounts for at least 20 per cent of congenital infections.

Transmission

is from urine, and possibly saliva. The virus can be acquired sexually. Acquired CMV in the newborn may result from transfusion with infected blood or ingestion of infected breast-milk.

Incubation period

is three weeks to three months.

Infectivity

can be prolonged.

Natural history

Congenital infection normally follows an asymptomatic maternal infection at any time during pregnancy. Only about 5 per cent of infected infants develop an acute illness at birth—cytomegalic inclusion disease (CID) associated with petechiae from thrombocytopaenia, hepatitis with jaundice, and microcephaly. Survivors may have features of cerebral palsy. Fewer than 10 per cent of infected infants will present with sensorineural deafness as the only consequence of infection. Acquired neonatal infection in the preterm infant may cause pneumonia and hepatitis, and has a significant mortality in the very low birthweight infant. Infection has occurred following the transfusion of blood from donors infected with CMV. Infection acquired by the term baby, or late in childhood and adolescence is relatively common but usually asymptomatic. Acquired infection does not cause deafness.

Diagnosis

Diagnosis of congenital CMV is best established by culture of urine or throat swabs within the first two weeks. It is not possible to distinguish between congenital and acquired infection in specimens cultured after this time.

Management and prevention

This is symptomatic as there is no effective antiviral agent. It is important to make an early diagnosis of sensorineural deafness (see rubella management p. 106). No immunization is available. Isolation from other children both within hospital and outside is not indicated and **carriers should not be excluded from nurseries**. There is little evidence that pregnant CMV sero-negative nurses are at increased risk of infection from babies secreting CMV. Nevertheless, nurses and day-care staff should exercise care with the secretions of all their charges and wash their hands after changing nappies. Donor blood for transfusion to the newborn is now routinely tested for CMV antibodies, and when there is evidence of recent infection this is withheld.

Diphtheria

Notifiable disease

Organism

Corynebacterium diphtheriae—a Gram-positive rod.

Epidemiology

The disease is now rare in developed countries because of routine immunization. It still causes considerable morbidity and mortality in the developing countries.

Transmission

is by droplet infection from nose and throat secretions. Unusual sites of infection, for example skin ulcers, may result from direct contact or be spread through fomites (see Glossary).

Incubation period

is 2–5 days but can be longer. Human beings are the only known reservoir of *C. diphtheriae*.

Period of infectivity

is two weeks or less, and under four days following antibiotic treatment.

Natural history

The disease usually presents as a membraneous nasopharyngitis or laryngotracheitis. For one to two days a sore throat and low-grade fever are associated with a spreading membrane in the throat that may cause respiratory obstruction (diphtheritic croup) and releases a powerful exotoxin that causes local tissue necrosis and attacks the myocardium of the heart and motor nerves: notably of the soft palate, eyes and diaphragm. The course of the illness depends on the severity of the toxaemia and the degree of immunity conferred by previous immunization. Milder infections in the partially immune may lead to uneventful recovery with the membrane sloughing off in 6–7 days. Severe infections occur in the unimmunized and are characterized by increasing toxaemia progressing to cardio-vascular collapse, stupor, coma, and death.

Diagnosis

Although diphtheria is a rare condition in the UK, cases still occur and the diagnosis must be considered in any membraneous condition of the throat, especially in children recently arrived from abroad, or their unimmunized contacts, and in those of doubtful immune status. Cultures should be taken from the nose and throat or from any site which may be contaminated (e.g. weeping skin ulcers). If possible, the swab should be taken from under the membrane. The laboratory should be consulted in advance as special media will be used to accelerate growth and thus identification of the organism.

Management

Children should be isolated and the antitoxin administered immediately the diagnosis is suspected. The dose is calculated according to the size of the membrane, the degree of toxicity, and the duration of illness. Antitoxin may be given im or iv depending on volume required and the severity of illness. Intradermal testing with 1:100 dilution is recommended prior to administration. Benzyl penicillin should be given intravenously. In cases of intermediate severity the potentially lethal complications must be anticipated.

Control measures

Close contacts, whether immunized or not, should have throat swabs, and carriers should be given a course of antibiotic. Contacts previously immunized should receive a booster dose of Diphtheria/Tetanus/Pertussis (DTP) or DT vaccine if not boosted in the previous five years. Close contacts not previously immunized should be given antibiotic prophylaxis (penicillin or erythromycin) and immunized.

Fifth disease/erythema infectiosum/slapped cheeks syndrome

Organism

Human parvovirus B19—a small DNA virus.

Epidemiology

Infection may occur in any month of the year but peaks occur in late winter, early spring.

Transmission

is by person-to-person spread by droplet infection from the respiratory tract. The virus may also be acquired through infected blood products (e.g. factor VIII concentrates).

Incubation period

is between seven and 22 days.

Infectivity

is high during the early stage of the illness with excretion of the virus from the respiratory tract.

Natural history

Fifth disease is a mild, acute illness occurring most often in children aged 5–14 years. There is a mild prodrome with fever and coryza. The rash is maculopapular and usually starts on the face as a bright red exanthem, hence the term 'slapped cheeks' syndrome. The rash spreads to the trunk and limbs where, on fading, it assumes a lace-like appearance. Constitutional symptoms are minimal: in children, associated respiratory symptoms are the most common feature; in adults, joint pain is a frequent occurrence. The diagnosis in sporadic cases is difficult and not easily differentiated from other exanthemous infections, especially rubella, whereas in community or school outbreaks the clustering of cases results in increased awareness and provides circumstantial support for the diagnosis.

Patients with inherited disorders of red cells can develop aplastic crises following infection with B19 human parvovirus because of temporary arrest of erythropoiesis. Infection in pregnancy may very occasionally result in hydrops fetalis.

Diagnosis

This is usually a clinical diagnosis. The virus is difficult to identify but serum IgM antibodies can be detected following infection.

Treatment

Symptomatic.

Gastrointestinal infections

Dysentery and typhoid fever are notifiable conditions

Epidemiology

Infections in the UK are normally mild, but may be severe in very young children and the immunosuppressed. Most cases of diarrhoea and vomiting in young children are caused by virus infection: rotavirus, astrovirus, adenovirus, and enterovirus. Bacterial causes of infection include *Salmonella* sp., *Campylobacter jejuni*, and *Yersinia enterocolitica*. *Shigella* sp. and *Vibrio cholerae* infection should be considered in children with severe diarrhoea who have been abroad. Enteropathic *Escherichia coli* infections of infancy are now rarely a cause of disease but outbreaks of verotoxic *E. coli* can cause a severe haemorrhagic colitis in all age groups. Food poisoning may follow ingestion of the exotoxins of *Bacillus cereus* and *Staphylococcus aureus*. The protozoans *Cryptosporidium* and *Giardia lamblia* are increasingly recognized as important causes of diarrhoea, especially in young children. Amoebic dysentery is only seen in children who have been abroad.

Transmission

of all these organisms is by the faecal–oral route, and, for viruses, the respiratory route as well. The incubation period and infectivity are variable (see Appendix 3).

Natural history

Viral infections are normally associated with diarrhoea and vomiting, and sometimes upper-respiratory-tract symptoms. Vomiting may precede diarrhoea in rotavirus infection. These infections are usually self-limiting and recovery occurs in 48–72 hours.

The bacterial infections normally present with diarrhoea and there is generally a systemic 'upset' with fever and headache. Dysentery (bloody, purulent diarrhoea) is a feature of *Shigella* sp. infections, which in young children may be associated with febrile convulsions. *Campylobacter jejuni* infection causes a systemic upset, abdominal pain, and frank blood may be passed in the stool. Similar symptoms may occur with *Yersinia enterocolitica* infection, which may mimic appendicitis or ulcerative colitis. Food poisoning is characterized by vomiting and diarrhoea, with onset a few hours after ingestion of the exotoxin.

Diagnosis

Both vomiting and diarrhoea may be features of other conditions such as meningitis, otitis media, urinary-tract infection, appendicitis, and intussusception. For a fuller discussion see p. 24.

In acute florid diarrhoea associated with a systemic illness both stool and blood should be sent for bacterial culture. Even with full investigation in hospital a pathogen is only identified in 80 per cent of cases; while in cases managed in the community the proportion is only 30 per cent. In more chronic diarrhoea, particularly in children, microscopy for ova and cysts becomes more important. Viral identification is possible by electron microscopy; however, this is a time-consuming investigation and consideration has to be given as to whether the result will affect management.

Management

Children with gastroenteritis are at risk of dehydration, and this always needs to be considered in any child with diarrhoea or vomiting. Appropriate treatment depends on an accurate assessment of the degree of dehydration (see Table 8). Children with less than 5 per cent dehydration may be able to remain at home. Those with over 5 per cent dehydration will need hospital admission.

If the diarrhoea is mild and there is no evidence of dehydration, the child can continue on a normal diet at home (breast milk, formula feed, or solids). There is no place at home or in hospital for antimotility drugs (opiates, loperamide) in the treatment of acute diarrhoea. Likewise, absorbent mixtures, such as chalk and kaolin, should not be used. Infants and children can become dehydrated quickly, and parents should be warned of the signs of this. Written advice is helpful for parents, advising them to watch for the signs of deterioration, such as worsening diarrhoea or vomiting, decreased frequency of wet nappies/urination, sleepiness, and sunken eyes.

Table 8 Signs of different degrees of dehydration

Sign	Less than 5% dehydration	More than 5% dehydration	More than 10% dehydration
Skin	Normal tension	Loss of turgor	Mottled, poor capillary return
Fontanelle (if open)	Normal	Depressed	Deeply depressed
Eyes	Not sunken	Sunken, reduced intraocular pressure	Sunken, reduced intraocular pressure
Lips	Moist	Dry	Dry
Peripheral pulses	Normal	Normal	Poor volume and tachycardia
Blood-pressure	Normal	Normal	Low
Behaviour	Unchanged	Lethargic	Prostation, coma
Urine output	Still wetting nappies or urinating at usual frequency	Long periods between micturition	Anuric

NB: Children with hypernatremic dehydration have a doughy feel to the skin and may not appear as dehydrated.

Where vomiting is troublesome, or diarrhoea is more severe, then a glucose electrolyte mixture containing sodium, potassium, chloride, bicarbonate, and glucose in water can be given (80–150 ml/kg/24 h, depending on age). If commercial preparations (Dioralyte, Rehidrat) are prescribed, it is essential to educate parents as to their correct use, to prevent incorrect reconstitution or their being employed as well as, rather than instead of, feeds. Small infants may become hypoglycaemic if such preparations are administered for more than a short period, and the advice of a paediatrician should be sought if no improvement has occurred within 24 hours of the start of the treatment.

Table 9 Treatment of dehydration

Example: a 10 kg infant with 10% dehydration—

(1) Treat shock with plasma:
20 ml/kg over first half hour = 200 ml

(2) Fluid deficit = 1 kg = 1000 ml
Aim to correct half deficit in first 8 hours, and half in next 16 hours:

First 8 hours: $\frac{500}{8}$ ml = 62 ml/h, then $\frac{500}{16}$ ml = 31 ml/h

(3) Aim to give maintenance fluid, i.e. 10 kg infant requires 100 ml/kg/day, so needs:

$\frac{1000}{24}$ = 43 ml/h

Thus, in first half hour, 200 ml plasma, then 105 ml (62 + 43)/h to 8 hours, and 74 ml (31 + 43)/h from 8–24 hours

---

In hospital, barrier nursing is required. When a child is less than 5 per cent dehydrated either normal fluid or an electrolyte mixture can be offered. If the child is drinking and dehydration is 5 per cent, an oral glucose electrolyte mixture should be given. If the symptoms fail to respond to oral rehydration, or there is inadequate intake or persistent vomiting, then intravenous rehydration is recommended. In the more severely dehydrated child, intravenous therapy should be started on admission to hospital. Plasma electrolytes must be measured and blood cultures should be collected at the same time. The child is weighed and the amount of fluid to be given is calculated as in Table 9.

Most infants in the UK have isotonic dehydration. If given one-fifth (0.18 per cent) normal saline as fluid replacement, hyponatraemia may develop, so initial rehydration should be with either normal or one-half normal saline with added dextrose to reduce the risk of hypoglycaemia. Hypernatraemic dehydration (plasma sodium more than 150 mmd/l) should be corrected more slowly using normal saline. Antibiotics may sometimes be given to treat systemic illness and shorten the period of infectivity, as shown in Table 10.

Table 10 Antibiotics given for specific gastrointestinal infections

Infection	Antibiotics
Campylobacter jejuni	In severe infection only, erythromycin 30 mg/kg/day, 3 times daily for 3 days
Entamoeba histolytica	Metronidazole. Dosage given in Appendix 2
Giardia lamblia	Metronidazole. Dosage given in Appendix 2
Salmonella typhi	Chloramphenicol 50 mg/kg/day oral, or 75 mg/kg/day iv, 4 times daily for 14 days; or ampicillin 100 mg/kg/day, 4 times daily for 14 days
Shigella dysentery	Ampicillin 100 mg/kg/day in 4 doses daily for 5 days, or co-trimoxazole 10 mg/kg/day as trimethoprin in 2 divided doses for 5 days
Vibrio cholerae	In children aged nine and under, co-trimoxazole as for Shigella; in children aged 10 and over, tetracycline 50 mg/kg/day 4 times daily for 2 days

Post-enteritis syndrome

This is characterized by continuing diarrhoea and is often associated with lactose intolerance, which can be diagnosed by testing the liquid portion of the stool for reducing sugars using Clinitest tablets (a value over 1 per cent is significant). Cows' milk protein intolerance may also develop. For both conditions a lactose-free soya milk (Cow & Gate formula S, Prosobee, Wysoy) may be prescribed by the paediatrician.

Guidelines for prevention of gastroenteritis in day-care facilities, schools, and the home

Special attention should be given to the following.

1. In making up formula feeds care must be taken that bottles are adequately sterilized and milk is not allowed to stand for long periods.

Table 11 A guide to exclusion of children from day care or school following gastroenteritis. Children should be excluded while symptomatic, although exclusion may be less strictly observed for secondary-school children. (Adapted from: *Notes on the control of human sources of gastrointestinal infections, infestation and bacterial intoxication in the United Kingdom.* Communicable Disease Report, Supplement 1, 1990.)

Organism	Criteria of clearance	Notifiable
Campylobacter	When diarrhoea ceases	No
Bacillary dysentery (Shigellosis)	3 negative faeces at least 24 hrs apart	Yes
Amoebic dysentery	3 negative faeces (for cysts)	Yes
E. coli (enteropathogenic strains)	3 negative faeces	No
Virus gastroenteritis Rotavirus Others	72 hours after diarrhoea ceases	No
Salmonellosis (excluding typhoid, paratyphoid)	3 negative faeces	Yes
Typhoid, paratyphoid	3 negative faeces	Yes
Giardiasis	None	No
Cryptosporidiosis	None	No

2. Ensure everyone (staff, parents, and children) understands the importance of handwashing with soap and hot water after using the toilet, changing nappies, and before preparing or eating food.

3. Toileting and nappy-changing areas must be well separated from food-preparation areas.

4. Where cases have occurred, children and staff with acute diarrhoea should be excluded for the duration of symptoms

where no organism is identified. Where a specific cause is identified, negative stool samples may need to be obtained before readmission (see Table 11). Exclusion may not always be necessary in schools where effective hygiene practices can be implemented. Decisions will depend on the organism and local facilities, and will be made in consultation with the designated medical officer.

5. Specimens may need to be taken from contacts of cases. However, the Medical Officer of Environmental Health (MOEH) will need to give advice as to when this is appropriate.
6. When there is a sudden outbreak involving several children, food poisoning must be considered and the MOEH involved immediately.
7. It will need to be explained to staff that most cases of childhood diarrhoea have a viral cause and stool cultures will be negative.

Glandular fever—infectious mononucleosis

Organism

Epstein–Barr virus (EBV) which is a herpes virus.

Epidemiology

Infection is often subclinical in infancy and childhood, but commonly produces illness in the adolescent and young adult, and most adults are seropositive, indicating that they have experienced a previous infection.

Transmission

is by saliva, with spread by close contact in young children. Glandular fever has been dubbed 'the kissing disease' because of the high incidence of clinical infection in late adolescence. Reactivation of EBV infection may occur in the immunosuppressed patient.

Incubation period

is between 30 and 50 days.

Infectivity

may be prolonged for several months following infection.

Natural history

The illness normally begins with fever, headache, and malaise, and is followed by a severe sore throat and lymphadenopathy. Fever may last from several days to two weeks. Lymphadenopathy is generalized but more pronounced in the glands of the neck. A white exudate is often present on the enlarged tonsils and petechiae may be seen on the palate. An erythematous maculopapular rash is seen frequently in children given ampicillin inappropriately for treatment of this infection. Splenomegaly can be detected in most patients and liver enlargement, sometimes associated with jaundice, although common, is a less consistent clinical finding. Uncommon complications include pneumonia, aseptic meningitis, and transverse myelitis. Pneumonia is a feature of EBV infection in children with AIDS.

Diagnosis

When tonsillitis, lymphadenopathy, and splenomegaly are seen together, infectious mononucleosis is the probable diagnosis. A rash developing after ampicillin prescribed for tonsillitis is often diagnostic of EBV infection.

Haematological changes in infectious mononucleosis are non-specific; there may be a leukopenia or a leucocytosis but there is normally an increase in 'atypical' lymphocytes. Patients develop a high titre of specific antibodies known as agglutinins because of their ability to cause sheep red blood cells to clump together. These are detected in the 'monospot' or 'Paul Bunnell' tests. However, these may not become positive until 3–4 weeks after the onset of symptoms.

Other conditions to be differentiated from infectious mononucleosis include streptococcal tonsillitis, diphtheria, viral hepatitis, and acquired cytomegalovirus infection. If recovery is delayed, it is important to exclude acute lymphoblastic leukaemia which may present with similar signs.

Treatment

This is symptomatic with analgesics and antipyretics. Indications for hospital admission include airway obstruction from large tonsils (more common in the young adult than child) or neurological complications. Isolation is not required and there is no quarantine period.

Gonococcal infections

Ophthalmia neonatorum is a notifiable disease

Organism

Neisseria gonorrhoeae which is a paired, Gram-negative coccus.

Epidemiology

This infection occurs only in humans. It is commonest amongst adults with multiple sexual partners.

Transmission

is by direct sexual contact, or to the infant during parturition causing ophthalmia neonatorum (a purulent discharge from the eye of an infant within 21 days of birth). Infection during childhood is almost certainly the result of sexual abuse, and cannot occur through other ways such as contact with an adult in a bath, from lavatory seats, or towels.

Incubation period

is 2–7 days.

Infectivity

continues until the disease is treated.

Natural history

Gonococcal ophthalmia neonatorum in the newborn normally develops as an acute purulent conjunctivitis 2–5 days after birth. Untreated, corneal scarring or even loss of the eye may follow. Spread to the joints or meninges may occur. Neonatal vaginitis has been reported but is rare. Infection in childhood may result in vulvovaginitis or urethritis, and after puberty in endocervicitis or pelvic inflammatory disease. Proctitis, pharyngitis, or conjunctivitis may be seen in all age groups.

Diagnosis

A Gram stain of the exudate should be performed immediately in the presence of purulent conjunctivitis. In many laboratories this is performed on a smear taken from a single swab which is also used for culture. Chlamydial conjunctivitis cannot be differentiated on clinical grounds, so it is advised to collect a specimen for chlamydial identification at the same time. Gonococcal culture may be indicated following sexual abuse or in a child with a vaginal or urethral discharge (see Table 3). *Chlamydia trachomatis* infection may produce similar symptoms in childhood. A serological test for syphilis should be considered where gonococcal infection is present.

Treatment

Treatment of ophthalmia neonatorum with systemic benzyl penicillin and saline washes to the eye should be started immediately following identification of Gram-negative cocci on Gram stain, or culture of *Neisseria gonorrhoeae*. In childhood gonococcal infection, a single injection of procaine penicillin, or oral ampicillin can be used. Amoxicillin and ampicillin are ineffective for anorectal infections and pharyngitis. Adolescents should also be treated with procaine penicillin. Penicillin resistance is unusual; children with a true penicillin allergy should be treated with spectinomycin and erythromycin. In neonatal infections the mother and father or consort should be referred to a genitourinary disease clinic. In older children, the local procedure for suspected sexual abuse must be initiated.

Haemolytic uraemic syndrome

This syndrome is relatively uncommon even in specialized hospital practice. However, its inclusion in this book is justified by the importance of early recognition and the confirmed association with infection caused by verocytotoxin producing strains of *Escherichia coli*, the apparent increase in incidence reflected in reports to the British Paediatric Surveillance Unit (BPSU). It is now the commonest cause of acute renal failure in childhood.

Organism

The exact cause is unknown. A recent study showed verocytotoxin producing strains in one-third of children with haemolytic uraemic syndrome. If stools were cultured within 3 days of the onset of diarrhoea culture was positive in 62 per cent of patients.

Epidemiology

There are small outbreaks but most cases occur sporadically. There can be a familial or genetic predisposition, with both autosomal recessive and dominant forms reported. The syndrome predominates in children under three years of age, has a mortality of 20 per cent, and there is significant chronic illness in some survivors.

Natural history

There is usually a well-defined prodromal illness such as gastroenteritis often with bloody diarrhoea. Fever is transient and mild but the child looks and feels ill with quite severe abdominal pain that may lead to referral to a surgical ward. Although the gastrointestinal symptoms and signs may settle after one or two days, the child's general condition remains poor and more specific features of the syndrome develop: haematuria and proteinuria with oliguria which may progress rapidly to anuria; hypertension; haemolytic anaemia with red-cell fragmentation and thrombocytopaenia prominent on a blood film; CNS signs such as alterations in consciousness and seizure activity.

The histo-pathological lesion is a widespread thrombotic micro-angiopathy with endothelial damage resulting either directly from a toxic agent or indirectly through mechanical interference with the microcirculation from fibrin deposition. In addition to the anaemia and thrombocytopaenia described above, plasma urea and creatinine are elevated. Depending on the stage of the illness there may be a decrease in clotting factors and an increase in fibrin-degradation products.

Management

As this syndrome has a significant mortality, intensive treatment should be started as soon as the condition is suspected. This is best achieved with specialized staff and facilities and frequent monitoring of vital signs, fluid and electrolyte balance, body weight, blood-pressure, and the early provision of peritoneal dialysis. Severe anaemia should be corrected by small transfusions of packed cells. Over-hydration is particularly dangerous and management is aided by establishing a central venous line. Broad-spectrum antibiotics, but not those potentially nephrotoxic, are usually given in the early stages of the syndrome as the presenting features are difficult to distinguish from those of severe infection, but there is no evidence that they are always necessary. Steroids are not indicated.

Although milder cases with oliguria may resolve spontaneously without dialysis, there is evidence that the early introduction of peritoneal dialysis may improve the outcome. Haemodialysis is rarely necessary but peritoneal dialysis may be required for several weeks before the gradual return of renal function. In survivors the majority of children go on to complete recovery, although, in a few there may be some residual renal insufficiency or hypertension.

Haemophilus influenzae infection

Organism

Haemophilus influenzae is a small, Gram-negative cocco-bacillus classified into capsular serotypes a–f and those without capsules.

Epidemiology

Haemophilus influenzae inhabits the upper respiratory tract and asymptomatic colonization is common with non-capsulated strains present in the throat of 60–90 per cent of individuals, and encapsulated strains in approximately 5 per cent. Most *H. influenzae* meningitis in the newborn is caused by non-typeable organisms; *H. influenzae* serotype b produces epiglottitis and meningitis in later infancy and childhood, with infection uncommon over the age of five. There is evidence from the USA that there is significantly increased risk of invasive infection among household contacts of index cases. This applies when the contacts are under the age of four. Outside the neonatal period, the non-typeable strains cause less severe illness, such as otitis media.

Transmission

is by inhalation of droplets of respiratory-tract secretions containing the organisms.

Incubation period

is not known, and difficult to establish because children may become colonized for some time before infection occurs.

Natural history

H. influenzae, is a major cause of meningitis from the neonatal period to the age of four. Epiglottitis is invariably caused by this organism and is most common from two to four years but can occur during later childhood and adult life (see p. 8). *H. influenzae* is also a cause of septic arthritis, cellulitis, bacteraemia, pneumonia, and empyema.

Diagnosis

For invasive infections, appropriate body fluids such as CSF, blood, or synovial fluid should be obtained for Gram stain and culture. Antigen detection in body fluids using latex agglutination or counter immunoelectrophoresis tests may be useful, especially in children who have received prior antibiotic treatment.

Management

Invasive infections such as meningitis and epiglottitis in infants and children over one month of age should be treated with ampicillin and chloramphenicol. For the neonate, ampicillin and an aminoglycoside or cephalosporin (e.g. cefotaxime) can be used. A single anti-microbial can be given once the results of sensitivity testing is available. Up to 10 per cent of invasive strains are resistant to ampicillin; chloramphenicol resistance is rare. It is recommended that a minimum of 7 days' treatment is given for cases of meningitis. Localized infections such as otitis media can usually be successfully treated with ampicillin but, in the case of resistant strains, alternative antibiotics include co-trimoxazole, amoxycillin/clavulanic acid, or cephaclor.

Chemoprophylaxis

When there is another child aged 3 or less in the house of a case of invasive type b infection, rifampicin prophylaxis is recommended for all household contacts. The index case should also receive rifampicin, since standard treatment does not eradicate nasopharyngeal carriage. Rifampicin is an enzyme inducer in the liver, and chloramphenicol plasma levels are lowered when both antibiotics are given together. Because of this it is advisable to give rifampicin towards the end of the course of treatment.

Prospects for immunization

A vaccine consisting of purified type b capsular polysaccharide is safe and effective in preventing invasive type b infections, but only in children of 24 months or older. This vaccine is recommended as a routine immunization in the USA where *H. influenzae* is more common, but is **not licensed for use in the UK**. Another vaccine which combines a polysaccharide and protein antigen has been given in the UK at the same time as the triple vaccine (the first dose at 3 months), and found to be effective.

Hand, foot, and mouth disease

Organism

Coxsackie virus—several different sub-types.

Epidemiology

This is a relatively common condition which tends to occur in epidemics and is not to be confused with foot-and-mouth disease which occurs in cattle. Infections predominate in the summer and autumn in pre-school children.

Transmission

is by droplets from the respiratory tract, by direct contact with the rash, and by the faecal–oral route.

Incubation period

is 3–5 days.

Infectivity

can be prolonged as the virus may remain in the stool for several weeks.

Natural history

The illness is characterized by vesicular lesions with a red base, which in the oral cavity are seen on the fauces, tongue, and side of the mouth. The rash is also seen on the hands and soles of the feet. There may be a history of low-grade fever for 4–6 days preceding the rash.

Diagnosis

This is on clinical grounds. Viral isolation is unnecessary.

Management

No treatment is needed. Because of the ease of spread amongst pre-school children they should be kept away from their peers until the lesions clear from the hands.

Hepatitis A (infective jaundice)

Notifiable disease

Organism

An enterovirus type 72.

Epidemiology

This is the commonest cause of jaundice in children.

Transmission

is via the faecal–oral route and also occurs through contamination of food or water as the virus is relatively resistant. Epidemics result from contamination with raw sewage. In children the disease is relatively mild with anicteric infection being common (approximately 80 per cent).

Incubation period

is 15–40 days.

Infectivity

is maximal during the latter half of the incubation period but disappears quickly following development of jaundice or other symptoms. Infection is commoner amongst children in poor social circumstances and in institutional care or other circumstances where hygiene or sanitation is poor.

Natural history

In symptomatic cases fever commonly precedes the onset of jaundice and is accompanied (with or without jaundice) by headache, anorexia, nausea, vomiting, and abdominal pain from a tender, enlarged liver. Once jaundice accompanied by dark urine appears the child may feel better, although return of appetite and full vigour is usually delayed until clearing of the jaundice in about two weeks. Convalescence is brief and full recovery the usual outcome. Extremely rarely a child may develop liver failure from fulminating hepatitis.

Diagnosis

Diagnosis is usually on clinical grounds. Urobilinogen can be detected in the urine at the onset of jaundice. Laboratory tests show a transient rise in serum transaminase levels for 1–3 weeks with a rise in bilirubin at the peak of transaminase disturbance. When the course of the illness appears to be more severe or prolonged than expected, hepatitis B infection should be excluded (see p. 74). Serological tests for IgG anti-HAV (hepatitis A virus) and IgM anti-HAV are available but rarely indicated.

Management

There is no specific treatment. Hospital admission is undesirable and rarely necessary. However, if this is unavoidable, the child should be nursed in a cubicle and enteric precautions taken. (These can be discontinued a few days after the jaundice appears—see Glossary.) The importance of personal hygiene in preventing spread should be emphasized to parents and other carers of children. Careful handwashing is essential after nappy-changing or toiletting and before preparing or serving food and drink. Children with undiagnosed jaundice should be managed with precautions applicable to both hepatitis A and B until a diagnosis is made. This means treating blood and body fluids as if hepatitis B positive. Close contacts can be given human normal immunoglobulin (HNIG): 250 mg for children up to the age of nine; 500 mg for children of 10 and over.

Hepatitis B

Notifiable disease

Organism

A DNA-containing virus 42 nm in diameter. The virus is a double-shelled particle with the outer surface component, the hepatitis B surface antigen (HBsAg) used as the marker which identifies the carrier state or chronic hepatitis B. Two other antigens of hepatitis B infection have also been identified—the core antigen (HBcAg) and the e antigen (HBeAg), the latter being used as a marker of infectivity. The disease is transmitted by the introduction through the skin or mucous membrane of blood or blood products containing the virus.

Epidemiology

Children at particular risk include those who receive frequent transfusions of blood or blood products, e.g. in haemophilia; those on chronic haemo-dialysis; infants born to mothers who are HBeAg positive and, to a lesser extent, those with mothers who are HBsAg positive without being 'e' positive. Because the prevalence of the carrier state varies so much according to racial group, the risk of perinatal transmission will also vary with ethnic origin. In Asia the risk to infants born to mothers of Chinese origin may be as high as 40 per cent, whereas in Caucasian mothers the carrier state is uncommon (0.1–0.2 per cent) and therefore perinatal transmission is extremely rare. It is, however, important to identify intravenous drug abusing mothers as a high-risk group. The virus does not cross the placenta and transmission from mother to child probably occurs during or just after birth from a leak of maternal blood into the infant's circulation or through a break in the skin or mucous membranes. Subclinical infection with the development of a chronic carrier state may occur in the child. There is a clear association between the carrier state, chronic liver disease, and the development of hepatocellular carcinoma in later life, particularly in non-Caucasians.

Incubation period

is usually 60–90 days but may be as long as six months.

Infectivity

is low unless there is blood-to-blood contact.

Natural history

Infection with hepatitis B virus usually results in an apparently mild illness with anorexia, nausea, and general malaise. A prodrome with arthralgia and a rash may occur. Obvious jaundice can develop but, as with hepatitis A, anicteric infection is common. Marked jaundice is unusual in children, although the serum bilirubin is usually elevated. Compared with hepatitis A, laboratory testing reveals a more prolonged disturbance of serum transaminases, usually for 30–60 days. Fulminant hepatitis occasionally occurs with onset of hepatic failure within four weeks after the onset of acute hepatitis. As with hepatitis A, the overall prognosis including the survival rate is influenced by age, being much better in children than in adults.

Hepatitis B is also associated with more lasting morbidity and about 10 per cent will develop evidence of chronic disease, either chronic persistent hepatitis or chronic active hepatitis. The chronic state may follow mild anicteric forms of hepatitis. Primary liver carcinoma is an established consequence in young adults following childhood infection, though this is commoner amongst individuals infected in Africa or Asia rather than in Europe.

Diagnosis

Serological testing for HBsAg is useful in diagnosis and for the detection of carriers. The presence of HBeAg indicates that an individual will be infectious, but if HBe antibody is also present, the infectivity will be low.

Management

There is no specific treatment for hepatitis B infection. As for hepatitis A, mild cases should be cared for in the home. Where hospitalization is required, infected children should be barrier nursed and precautions taken in handling blood and other body fluids. Patients with undiagnosed jaundice should be managed with precautions applicable to both hepatitis A and B until the aetiology is established. Infants born to HBsAg positive mothers do not need to be isolated but care should be taken with blood/body fluids because 1–2 per cent will have become infected by perinatal transmission. They will require immunization, and this is essential if the mother is e antigen positive (see p. 166). Gloves should be worn by staff undertaking procedures involving the handling of blood or body fluids of these patients.

Herpes simplex

Organism

This is a DNA virus. Type 1 (HSV1) is a cause of cold sores and encephalitis in childhood, and type 2 (HSV2) is the cause of most neonatal infection.

Neonatal infection

Epidemiology

This occurs in approximately one per 50 000 live births. Most cases are associated with primary infection of the genital tract with HSV2.

Transmission

is by a maternal viraemia, by an ascending route to the uterus or during passage down the birth canal. The risk of infection following vaginal delivery in the presence of primary infection in the mother is about 50 per cent, but less than 8 per cent for recurrent infection.

Infectivity

is low (see Management).

Natural history

Infection may present as a generalized systemic illness with hepatitis and encephalitis; as localized central nervous system disease; or as localized infection of the skin, eyes, or mouth. The mortality is high with systemic disease.

Diagnosis

This is by tissue culture of secretions but a positive result may take three days. Rapid techniques using direct fluorescent antibody are being developed at present. Serology has no place in the diagnosis of acute infection.

Prevention and management

Because most cases result from a primary maternal infection where the history is short, diagnosis and treatment in the newborn are often delayed until many hours after onset of symptoms. It is current practice to perform regular viral culture on genital-tract secretions in women with known HSV infection during the last few weeks of pregnancy, so that Caesarean section can be undertaken early in labour if genital lesions are present. However, because of the delay in obtaining positive cultures and since most neonatal infection follows undiagnosed infection in the mother, this practice is of limited usefulness.

HSV infection in the newborn is treated with acyclovir; morbidity and mortality are reduced by treatment, in both neurological and generalized disease. Many paediatricians recommend treatment of all infants born to mothers with primary infection. Because of the low risk in association with recurrent maternal infection, it is recommended that infants born to such mothers are observed for at least 10 days after delivery and only treated when symptomatic.

The infected mother can nurse her own baby but needs to be kept in isolation from other infants. Because the risk of infection from attendants is extremely low, nurses with cold sores should be allowed to work provided lesions are covered and scrupulous attention is paid to handwashing.

Childhood infection

Epidemiology

Infections are common in childhood but most are minor.

Transmission

is by direct spread from infected lesions.

Incubation period

is 2–12 days.

Infectivity

following primary HSV1 can be prolonged for several weeks.

Natural history

Gingivostomatitis (infection of the gums and mouth) is the commonest significant manifestation of type 1 infection, presenting with fever and painful vesicles in the affected area. Infections in children with eczema may result in Kaposi's varicelliform eruption (eczema herpeticum) which may be complicated by bacterial infection. The lesions are similar to those seen in zoster (shingles) but are not restricted to the dermatome distribution (see Glossary). Where herpetic lesions are seen in the genital tract in childhood, they are almost certainly the result of sexual abuse and usually are due to HSV2. Encephalitis results from HSV type 1 and is usually a primary infection; it presents with altered consciousness and convulsions, and has a 50 per cent mortality.

Diagnosis

Because of the serious nature of both eczema herpeticum and encephalitis, a clinical diagnosis is sufficient for treatment to be started. The virus can be identified in tissue culture, by electron microscopy; rapid diagnostic methods are being introduced. Only rarely is virus identified in the CSF in encephalitis.

Treatment

The systemic antiviral agent, acyclovir, is the treatment of choice and should be given without delay in severe infections.

Influenza

Organism

The influenza viruses are orthomyxoviruses of three antigenic types (A, B, and C) but epidemic disease is caused by types A and B. In contrast to most other viruses, influenza A and B (especially A) constantly alter their antigenic substructure—antigenic 'drift'. This limits the effectiveness of vaccines from year to year and these have to be frequently modified to fit the components of the prevalent strains.

Epidemiology

The highest attack rates occur in school-age children, with secondary spread to adults and younger children in the household. Attack rates depend on the immunity conferred by previous infections or immunization. New strains occurring through antigenic drift may cause widespread epidemics which occur particularly in the winter, lasting 1–2 months.

Transmission

is by airborne droplets and through articles such as handkerchiefs recently contaminated by nasopharyngeal secretions.

Incubation period

is 1–3 days.

Infectivity

is high for 24 hours before symptoms appear, and for 24–48 hours thereafter.

Natural history

There is a wide spectrum of severity. Rapid onset of fever with rigors is accompanied by headache, diffuse muscle aches, and a dry cough. More widespread signs of respiratory infection may then follow including nasal congestion, a painful throat, stridor, and signs of lower-respiratory-tract involvement, including pneumonia, which is particularly likely to develop in children suffering from chronic cardiac or respiratory disease. In young infants influenza may mimic generalized sepsis with relatively few localizing respiratory signs. Although influenza alone can produce a severe respiratory illness, secondary bacterial invasion of the lungs with such organisms as *Staphylococcus aureus* and *Klebsiella pneumoniae* is particularly dangerous. Otitis media is another common bacterial complication. Viral complications such as myocarditis and encephalitis are seen in adults but are rarely a problem in childhood.

Diagnosis

Rapid diagnosis is rarely necessary but is possible through identification of the influenza antigen in nasopharyngeal secretions by immunofluorescent techniques or enzyme-linked immunosorbent assay (ELISA). Serological diagnosis is possible retrospectively by demonstrating a rise in antibody between acute and convalescent sera.

Treatment

Treatment is symptomatic in previously healthy individuals.

Control measures

It is recommended that children of all ages with cystic fibrosis should be immunized annually against the prevalent strain. Similarly, immunization should be considered for other children who may be at risk of severe infection, such as those with chronic lung and heart diseases.

Kawasaki disease—mucocutaneous lymph node syndrome (MCNLS)

Report to British Paediatric Surveillance Unit (BPSU)

Organism

Unknown. An infectious agent is suspected but none has been identified consistently to date.

Epidemiology

First described in Japan (1967) where the incidence is particularly high at about one in every 1000 children. The disease is now recognized world-wide. Over 100 cases were reported in 1987 to the BPSU but under-diagnosis and under-reporting remain. The vast majority of cases occur in children under five years with a peak occurrence at 1–2 years. The male : female ratio is 1.6 : 1.

Transmission

is unknown but even close childhood contacts do not seem to be at any increased risk.

Natural history

The illness begins with an abrupt onset of fever which may persist for 5–15 days, or even longer in some cases, and is unresponsive to antibiotics. After 2–3 days of unexplained fever, the characteristic features of the disease develop in succession and should suggest the diagnosis. These are:

(1) red eyes from inflamed conjunctivae;

(2) changes in the mouth—red, swollen lips which progress to cracking and fissuring after several days, strawberry tongue, pharyngeal erythema;

(3) rash: generalized erythematous eruption which may be punctate or maculo-papular;

(4) cervical lymphadenopathy—non-suppurative and may be unilateral;

(5) changes in fingers and toes—reddening, oedema, with desquamation on the tips after 2–3 weeks.

Resolution of fever with obvious improvement in the child's condition may have occurred by the time desquamation occurs, but fretfulness and anorexia may persist for several weeks. Other features in some patients include diarrhoea, arthritis, and arthralgia; aseptic meningitis, pneumonia, and a sterile pyuria. The most worrying feature of Kawasaki disease is occasional cardiac and coronary artery involvement. Routine echo-cardiography or angiography have demonstrated abnormalities of the coronary arteries ranging from mild dilatation or tortuosity to aneurysm formation in about 20 per cent of patients. Aneurysms are particularly frequent under the age of six months and may first appear 2–3 weeks after the onset of the illness. They usually regress but there is a mortality rate of 1–2 per cent usually from coronary artery thrombosis with myocardial infarction. Although there may be ECG changes (e.g. lengthening of QT_c interval, Twave flattening, and depression of S-T segments) aneurysm formation can occur without any ECG abnormality.

Diagnosis

There is no specific test for Kawasaki disease. Diagnosis is based on the complex of characteristic clinical and laboratory features occurring after several days of unexplained fever. The most useful test findings are a thrombocytosis of over 450 000 and often exceeding 1 000 000 mm^3 by the second or third week of the disease; a raised erythrocyte sedimentation rate (ESR), a leucocytosis of over 15 000 mm^3; elevated C-reactive protein and alpha-2 globulin. Many other diseases produce rashes, mucocutaneous lesions, and lymphadenopathy, but rarely as many as four of the five characteristic clinical features described above. Frequently confused with Kawasaki disease, especially in the first few days of the illness, are measles, scarlet fever, glandular fever, roseola infantum, and the systemic form of juvenile chronic arthritis (Still's disease).

Management

Isolation is unnecessary. With the possible exception of immunoglobulin (see below) there is no specific treatment which can prevent the potentially serious complications such as coronary artery involvement, carditis, and arthritis. Aspirin has been shown to reduce the risk of complications. It is administered initially in anti-inflammatory doses of 80–100 mg/kg/day in four divided doses. Once the fever has settled, the dose is reduced to 3–5 mg/day in one dose in order to decrease platelet adhesiveness. Low-dose aspirin treatment is continued for at least three months. If an aneurysm has been detected, aspirin therapy is recommended until the aneurysm resolves, which may take many months. Control trials from both the USA and Japan show a beneficial effect of intravenous gammaglobulin when given within 10 days of onset of illness (400 mg/kg dose, for 4 days). Corticosteroid drugs are contraindicated.

Listeriosis

Organism

Listeria monocytogenes is a gram-positive rod.

Epidemiology

L. monocytogenes is found in cattle, other animals, and silage. It has been isolated from unpasteurized soft cheeses, paté, salads, and microwave-ready meals. Outbreaks of infection have been traced to pasteurized soft cheese contaminated during processing. There has been a recent increase in neonatal infection in the United Kingdom. In the first 6 months of 1989 there were 152 reports of listeriosis to the CDSC, and about half of these were of maternal or neonatal infection.

Transmission

Transplacentally when the mother has an acute infection. *L. monocytogenes* may colonize the genital tract so that the infant may acquire the organism during delivery. Ten per cent of neonatal infections result from cross-infection.

Natural history

Congenital infection may result in stillbirth, or a septicaemic illness, normally within 48 hours of delivery. The liquor may be meconium stained, and infants may develop respiratory distress from pneumonia. Meningitis may occur, and careful examination of the pharynx may reveal red spots, or roseoles, which are characteristic of listeria infection.

Illness presenting later in the neonatal period takes the form of meningitis, which has a less acute onset and a lower mortality.

Diagnosis

Early onset infection may be characterized by leucopenia. Blood and cerebrospinal fluid (CSF) should be sent for culture. With the later onset meningitis, either neutrophils or mononuclear cells may predominate in CSF.

Treatment

Ampicillin (or penicillin) and gentamicin should be used for listeriosis. Because of the recent increase in such infection, a penicillin should be included in the treatment of any infant with suspected congenital bacterial infection prior to the result of culture. The cephalosporins are ineffective in this condition.

Prevention

Although the link between sporadic cases of listeriosis and isolation from foodstuffs has not been proven, pregnant women are advised to avoid unpasteurized cheese, paté, prewashed salads, and ensure that microwave-ready meals are adequately cooked.

Malaria

Notifiable disease

Organism

Plasmodium species (*falciparum, ovale, vivax, malariae*)—a protozoan.

Epidemiology

Imported malaria has increased dramatically in the seventies and eighties (Fig. 3); between 200 and 300 cases in children under 16 are now notified annually in England and Wales. The disease is endemic in Africa (except on the Mediterranean coast), the Indian subcontinent (ISC), the tropical Far East, South and Central America but not the West Indian Islands (except Haiti). Over half the UK cases are now travellers from the ISC (mainly vivax malaria) but there has been a recent upsurge in those from Africa (mainly the more serious falciparum variety).

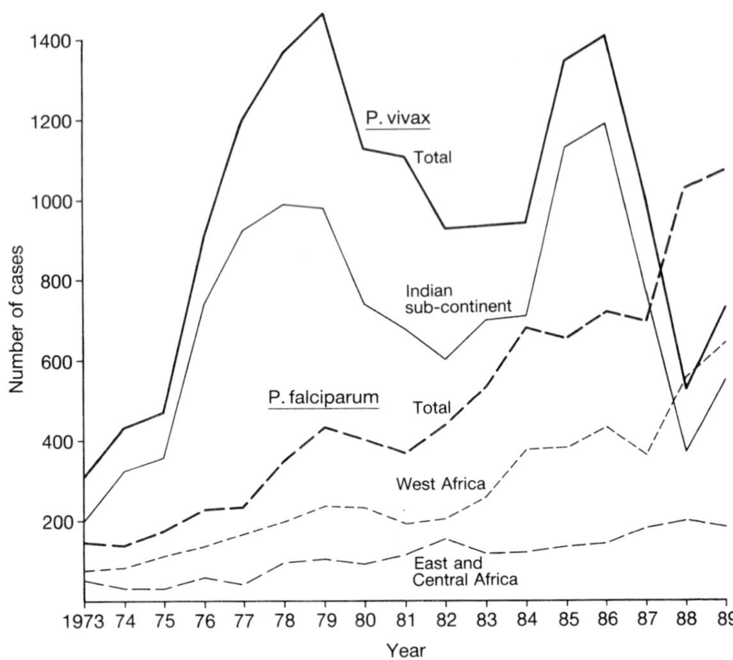

Fig. 3 Malaria Reference Laboratory Data, UK 1973–89. By courtesy of CDSC.

Transmission
is by the *Anopheles* mosquito and does not occur within the UK.

Incubation period
is 6–16 days, depending on the species; because the symptoms can be mild the child may present months after leaving the endemic area.

Natural history

The infected child typically has an intermittent fever with rigors and sweats which may occasionally progress to a convulsion and neurological involvement (cerebral malaria). Late and persistent symptoms are less common in children but do occur; they include nausea, jaundice, arthralgia, abdominal and back pain. Signs of malaria in infants may be non-specific with loss of appetite, irritability, and lethargy. Where infection has been frequent the child may be anaemic with splenomegaly. Congenital infection has been seen in the UK, usually amongst mothers born in the UK who have visited endemic areas.

Diagnosis

This is by a thick blood film which requires a fresh specimen sent promptly (with warning) to an experienced person. If antimalarials have been taken, these must be specified along with the country of travel.

Management

In most parts of the world *P. falciparum* is resistant to chloroquine, hence where this is the causative organism or the *Plasmodium* species is unknown treatment should be with quinine or mefloquine rather than chloroquine. Children with cerebral malaria, which has a high mortality, should be treated by physicians with experience of this disease.

Prevention is better than cure. For protection when travelling abroad see p. 230.

Measles

Notifiable disease

Organism

Measles virus, an RNA-containing virus in the paramyxovirus family.

Epidemiology

Because immunization falls short of targets in the UK, this disease is both endemic and epidemic (Fig. 4). It is uncommon under the age of one, because of protection from maternal antibody. The peak incidence is at school entry when infection is almost completely confined to unimmunized children. In the decade 1976–85, 165 children died from measles in the UK.

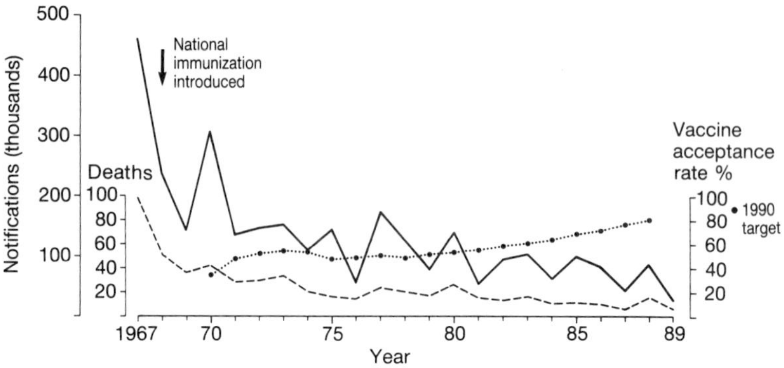

Fig. 4 Annual notifications, deaths, and vaccine acceptance rates for measles, England and Wales 1967–89. By courtesy of CDSC.

Transmission

is by airborne droplet spread (coughing and sneezing), from freshly soiled handkerchiefs, or by direct contact.

Incubation period

is 10 days (range 8–13).

Infectivity

is high. Children are infectious from shortly before the first symptoms to four days after the rash appears. They are most infectious prior to the appearance of the rash. In a highly susceptible population one case will, on average, cause 15 others. In a school this can mean 30–40 per cent of unimmunized children, in the home 70 per cent.

Natural history

Initially, the child develops coryzal symptoms which are followed by conjunctivitis causing photophobia and a dry cough. The tonsils may be red and Koplik's spots (like grains of salt) appear on the inside of the cheeks beside the molar teeth. After 2–3 days the temperature peaks and the rash appears first behind the ears then spreading over the face and down the body. The rash is more confluent over the upper part of the body. (For timing of signs see Fig. 2, p. 14.) Koplik's spots fade on the fifth or sixth day. If complications do not occur the temperature also returns to normal and the child feels better, though the cough may persist for another week. Most school-age children will, on average, miss a week of school with measles.

Complications are common and include croup in the prodromal period, viral or bacterial pneumonia, otitis media and conductive and sensorineural deafness, enteritis, encephalopathy, fits, and more severe CNS disease which can be fatal or cause brain damage. A late complication is subacute sclerosing panencephalitis (SSPE) occurring 5–10 years after infection. This is a slow, untreatable degenerative disease of the nervous system which is always handicapping and fatal in approximately 50 per cent of cases. The rate of complications of any kind amongst notified cases of measles is 1 in 10, while 1 in 70 children with the disease are admitted to hospital. Encephalopathy (including fits) occurs in 1 case in 500, and death in 1 case in 5000. Measles is also the most important cause of severe morbidity and mortality in immunosuppressed children being treated for malignant disease.

Diagnosis

Diagnosis is based on history and clinical signs. Many other rashes may be incorrectly diagnosed as measles unless the whole pattern of symptoms is considered.

Management

The child with uncomplicated disease needs nursing and temperature control rather than medication, other than paracetamol. It is traditional to darken the room, but most children will simply turn away from the light. Complications should be treated appropriately. Admission to hospital should be avoided where possible because of the risk to immunosuppressed children. There is no place for antibiotics unless there is clear evidence of bacterial infection, which, if it occurs, takes place late in the course of the disease.

Control measures

1. Isolation. This is indicated for four days after the appearance of the rash. The risk to immunosuppressed children should be considered. (For management in this group see below.)

2. Immunization (see p. 172). If live measles virus vaccine is given within 72 hours of exposure, it may lessen the disease in that child.
3. Immune globulin. Human normal immunoglobulin (HNIG) should be given to immunosuppressed children in contact with measles, preferably within 3 days of exposure. The dose is as follows: under 1 year 250 mg, 1–2 years, 500 mg; 3 and over 750 mg.

Family education

Many of the public and even some members of the nursing and medical profession believe that measles is a trivial illness. This has led to inadequate vaccine uptake and allowed disproportionate concern about vaccine reactions. A useful health-education device is the description by the author Roald Dahl of his daughter Olivia's death from measles. It is available in written form by sending a stamped addressed envelope to: Sandwell Health Authority, 8 Grange Road, West Bromwich, West Midlands B70 8PD.

Meningococcal disease

Notifiable—as meningitis or septicaemia alone
Meningitis is a notifiable condition

Organism

Neisseria meningitidis is a Gram-negative diplococcus. There are nine serotypes (A, B, C, D, X, Y, Z, 29-E, and W-135). Groups B and C are currently the most prevalent in the UK.

Epidemiology

Trends in the occurrence of meningococcal disease have shown periodic upsurges (e.g. 1940–5, the mid-seventies, and 1986–8.) *N. meningitidis* is currently the commonest cause of bacterial meningitis among children in the UK, mostly in the pre-school population. In 1988 there were 864 notified cases of meningococcal meningitis among children in England and Wales.

Transmission

occurs from person to person from naso-pharyngeal droplets or respiratory secretions. Infection may also develop in children and adults who have been carriers, and they may spread the disease, particularly to their close contacts.

Incubation period

is variable because infection may follow colonization. Treatment of invasive disease does not always result in eradication of the organism from the nasopharynx.

Natural history

The reasons why this organism suddenly invades a particular individual are not well understood. Onset of meningococcal bacteraemia or meningitis may be abrupt, with fever, rigors, and prostration. A petechial rash (sometimes preceded by a maculopapular rash) progressing to widespread and extensive bleeding into the skin (purpura) is characteristic of the more severe cases in which death may occur within a few hours. In convalescence, the purpuric lesions may slough (purpura necrotica). Pneumonia, unsuspected bacteraemia, arthritis, infective endocarditis, and chronic meningococcaemia are other less common invasive infections caused by this organism. Disease occurs at all ages but is most common in children under five years of age.

Diagnosis

Cultures of blood and cerebrospinal fluid are most useful in establishing the diagnosis. The organism may also be cultured from skin lesions and, rarely, synovial fluid. Rapid diagnosis may also be afforded through latex-agglutination tests which detect group-specific antigens in body fluids (e.g. CSF, urine).

Management

Treatment of invasive infections should be with intravenous benzyl penicillin. All strains are extremely sensitive to penicillin so that short courses of antibiotics are acceptable; treatment may be discontinued 48 hours after the child becomes apyrexial. Chloramphenicol should be combined with penicillin in children with meningitis until culture confirms meningococcal infection.

Children in whom meningococcal infection is suspected, especially in the presence of a petechial rash, should be given penicillin by their GP before transfer to hospital, particularly when the journey is a long one. Intravenous injection is preferred to intramuscular administration.

All household and day-care or school contacts should receive rifampicin, as should the index case, irrespective of whether meningococci can be isolated from the nasopharynx. Such prophylaxis should be given to contacts as soon as possible after a definite diagnosis has been made. Medical staff involved in mouth-to-mouth resuscitation should also be treated.

Vaccination should be considered when a cluster of cases occurs (apart from infections caused by B serotypes). It is now recommended that family members are immunized when a case occurs in the household. Vaccines against groups A, C, Y, and W-135 are available (C on a named-patient basis), but that to group A is less effective under the age of two and ineffective during the first few months. Group C vaccine does not produce immunity in children less than 2 years old. Many recent cases have been caused by B serotypes for which there is no immunization available. A new B vaccine is being evaluated at present.

Molluscum contagiosum

Organism

A poxvirus.

Epidemiology

A common infection which most individuals have at some time. Since lesions may be innocuous and then resolve, this mild infection is frequently missed.

Transmission

is by direct contact, the incubation period is from two to seven weeks, and infectivity is low.

Natural history

The virus results in a characteristic pearly papule with an obvious central dimple. Size varies from 1 to 5 mm. These can occur anywhere in children, most commonly in small crops due to direct contact. They will always resolve eventually, usually within nine months.

Diagnosis

Diagnosis is clinical.

Management

'Anti-wart' solutions available from chemists are ineffective. More drastic local treatments are not justified since the lesions will resolve spontaneously. If they occur in the child's genital or perianal area the possibility of sexual abuse should be considered. However, lesions may have spread to those areas from a child's hands.

Mumps

Notifiable disease

Organism

The mumps virus.

Epidemiology

This is endemic and common in the UK. Infections occur throughout childhood but are unusual in the first year of life. By adulthood most individuals have been infected. Complications of mumps infection result in the admission of approximately 1400 people (all ages) to hospital in the UK each year. Congenital abnormality following maternal infection is extremely rare.

Transmission

is by airborne droplet spread.

Incubation period

is 16–20 days.

Infectivity

is high, lasting from six days before to four days after swelling of the glands.

Natural history

The symptoms of mumps include headache, fever, and malaise followed by painful swelling of the parotid and/or submandibular salivary glands. The enlargement may be unilateral and asymmetrical. Illness is subclinical in approximately 30 per cent of infections. Complications are relatively common and include meningo-encephalitis (sometimes as the presenting feature), pancreatitis, deafness, and painful involvement of the testes and ovaries in adult sufferers. Meningoenchalitis induced by mumps vaccine is very rare. Such cases were brought into the BPSU scheme in 1990.

Diagnosis

In its classical form, mumps is unmistakable. Other organisms may cause a parotitis or nearby lymph-node enlargement. Antibody tests are available but seldom needed.

Management

This is symptomatic with analgesics where required. Only children with severe complications need to be admitted to hospital, where they should be isolated from immunosuppressed children, although even in this group the illness is rarely severe.

Nits (*Pediculosis capitis*)

Organism

Pediculus humanus capitis (head louse).

Epidemiology

This infestation is more common in areas of poverty, but nits are found amongst all social classes. Both nits (eggs) and lice are found in the hair.

Transmission

is by direct contact. The eggs take about nine days to hatch.

Infectivity

is high between household contacts and play-mates. The louse seems to be less common in Afro-Caribbean hair, it is thought because the different shape of the hair shaft makes nit attachment more difficult.

Natural history

After hatching the larva grows to maturity in nine days. It then feeds by sucking blood from the scalp and lays eggs (nits) which are cemented to the base of the hair shaft. The symptoms are an itchy scalp, though the child may not complain where infestation is light.

Diagnosis

The tenacious eggs stuck to the hair shaft are unmistakable; however the inexperienced observer may misidentify dandruff as nits, or vice versa.

Management

Two agents are active against head lice: malathion (Prioderm or Derbac) and carbaryl (Carylderm). Both should be applied as lotions to dry hair, and allowed to dry naturally (hair dryers will inactivate the drug). The hair should not be washed for 12 hours. The hair needs combing to remove nits. Lotions should be used where possible because they are alcohol based and kill both head lice and their eggs. The water-based shampoos are recommended in children under the age of three, and those with severe eczema or psoriasis. Because shampoos do not kill eggs, a second application has to be given at 7–10 days. They should be applied with warm, and not hot water, which may inactivate the insecticide. The hair of close contacts should be examined and treated. Many areas operate a policy of rotating malathion and carbaryl treatment every few years to prevent drug resistance developing.

Children with nits or lice do not need to be excluded from school unless their parents refuse treatment.

Routine screening of school populations by nurses is very time-consuming and is of no value. Parents should be encouraged to comb their own hair and that of their children twice daily; lice with broken legs do not survive. They should also check the hair of family members for nits weekly.

Pneumococcal infections

Organism

Streptococcus pneumoniae, a Gram-positive coccus. Also known as the pneumococcus.

Epidemiology

This is the usual cause of lobar pneumonia and common cause of acute pleural effusion in childhood. Many individuals are carriers of the organism in the upper respiratory tract; disease occurs in association with a viral upper-respiratory-tract infection or in the presence of a particularly virulent strain. Certain groups of children are at high risk of severe and sometimes fatal infection. These include children with nephrotic syndrome, sickle-cell anaemia, or after splenectomy. Patients with congenital or acquired immunodeficiency are also at risk.

Transmission
is from droplets of respiratory-tract secretions or recently soiled handkerchiefs.

Incubation period
is 1–3 days.

Infectivity
is low in most cases and isolation is not required.

Natural history

Pneumococcal pneumonia is normally lobar. Infection in the right upper lobe may be associated with meningism, and lower-lobe infection with abdominal pain. *Streptococcus pneumoniae* is a cause of meningitis (which may occur from the neonatal period into adulthood) and acute otitis media. Septicaemia may occur in the immunodepressed and in children with functional asplenia. Recurrent episodes of meningitis suggests chronic leakage of CSF.

Diagnosis

This is by identification of Gram-positive diplococci on Gram stain of secretions or following culture. Blood cultures may be helpful, and a polymorphonuclear leucocytosis is characteristic. Rapid diagnostic antigen-detection tests are available (latex-agglutination) but there is no evidence that they are any more sensitive than culture methods.

Treatment

Benzyl penicillin is the drug of choice for severe infections in childhood, with a minimum of 7 days for meningitis, and longer courses required in the presence of effusions or in the high-risk groups. Phenoxymethyl penicillin (penicillin V) is the drug of choice for lobar pneumonia in childhood. So close is the association with *S. pneumoniae* that treatment should be started before identification of the organism, although appropriate specimens should be collected for culture first (blood for culture and antigen detection, throat swab). Because of the poor absorption of oral penicillin, some clinicians prefer to give an initial dose of benzyl penicillin by intramuscular or intravenous injection. Where there is a clear history of penicillin allergy (rare in childhood) erythromycin can be given. Isolation is unnecessary.

Prevention

Children in the risk groups should be given anti-pneumococcal vaccine (Pneumovax) and prophylactic penicillin (see section on Special children, p. 216).

Poliomyelitis

Notifiable disease

Organism

Poliovirus, an enterovirus of three main types: 1, 2, and 3.

Epidemiology

A viral illness now eliminated from the UK, although imported or vaccine-associated cases may occur. It is endemic in many developing countries, especially the Indian subcontinent where annual incidence rates are estimated at 10–30 per 100 000 population. Because of the success of routine immunization, wild virus is rare in Britain and the majority of the few clinical cases now result from reversion of attenuated forms of the live vaccine, which can affect either the child being immunized or its unimmunized close contacts. From 1970 to 1984 only 70 definite cases, with two fatalities, were reported amongst residents of England and Wales.

Transmission

is by the faecal–oral route; food and water contamination is extremely rare and maintained swimming pools do not offer any risk.

Incubation period
is 7–14 days for paralytic cases.

Infectivity
via the faeces may be prolonged for six weeks or longer but is highest in the few days around the onset of symptoms.

Natural history

In children, cases are often subclinical or simply show as a mild febrile illness. However, wild or reverted attenuated virus can invade the nervous system causing meningitis or selectively attacking the motor cells in the spinal cord causing paralysis which can be permanent or fatal. Adults are more at risk of such complications.

Management

There is no specific treatment for the paralytic form apart from bed rest in the acute phase. It is essential to ensure that all individuals in contact are themselves immunized.

Rabies

Notifiable disease

Organism

A rhabdovirus.

Epidemiology

This disease is endemic in the animal population in most developing countries and much of Europe. Only six cases were notified in England and Wales between 1977 and 1987; three of those were in children bitten by dogs in the Indian subcontinent.

Transmission
is by bite, or lick of broken skin, by a rabid animal.

Incubation period
is 2–8 weeks. The more severe the bite and the closer the distance between the site of the bite and the brain, the shorter the incubation period.

Natural history

The child will present with fever followed by a deteriorating neurological status including anxiety, confusion, convulsions, and death. There will be a history of exposure to a rabid animal (usually lethal in the animal).

Diagnosis

Where possible, the suspect animal should be killed and brain samples tested for the virus. If the animal is still healthy two weeks after the bite/lick, there is no rabies risk. Specimens from the child (isolation of virus from saliva or CSF) rarely provide more than confirmation of a clinical diagnosis obvious by the deteriorating state.

Management

(See Travel abroad, pp. 236, 241.)

Respiratory syncytial virus (RSV) infection

(See bronchiolitis, p. 9.)

Organism

This is an RNA, paramyxovirus.

Epidemiology

Infections are most severe in the first few months of life. Infants at particular risk of severe infection are preterm, or with congenital heart disease. Smoking by one or more parents appears to increase susceptibility to infection. Infection occurs in epidemics normally in winter and spring, at a time when the highest rates of the sudden infant death syndrome are recorded, suggesting a possible role of this virus in its aetiology.

Transmission

is from respiratory-tract secretions, and man is the only source of infection. It has been shown that the virus may remain viable for up to six hours in secretions outside the body.

Incubation period

is 5–8 days.

Infectivity

lasts about seven days from onset of symptoms.

Natural history

This is the most important cause of bronchiolitis during infancy. In the preterm infant, signs may be non-specific and include lethargy and apnoea. In the term infant, signs are more localized to the respiratory system, with rapid breathing, intercostal recession and over-inflation of the upper chest. Auscultation with a stethoscope reveals crackles and wheezes. Complications include respiratory and cardiac failure.

Diagnosis

Nasopharyngeal aspirates can be sent to the laboratory early in the course of the infection for either culture or a rapid diagnostic procedure such as immunofluorescence, which has a higher sensitivity.

Management

Most infants with bronchiolitis can be managed at home. With more serious infection, hospital admission may be required for observation and tube feeding. Measurements of arterial gases may be required; hypoxia should be corrected with oxygen. A rising carbon dioxide level is a warning that intermittent positive-pressure ventilation may be necessary. Fluids should be restricted and electrolytes carefully monitored in severely ill infants. Diuretics should be used if heart failure develops. A newly developed anti-viral agent, ribavirin, has been shown to produce a marginal improvement in severely affected infants with congenital heart disease or bronchopulmonary dysplasia, and may be indicated in this group. This has to be administered as an aerosol and is extremely expensive (£600 for a three-day course). Infants should be isolated and careful handwashing employed to prevent spread to other hospitalized infants.

Prevention

Attempts at preparation of a vaccine have been unsuccessful.

Ringworm (Tinea)

Organism

Various fungal organisms of species *Microsporum* and *Trichophyton.*

Epidemiology

A widespread slow or chronic infection occurring in four clinical forms (see Natural history), some of which (scalp and body ringworm) may be acquired from animals.

Transmission

is by direct or indirect contact with infected lesions, including skin or hairs which have been shed. Hence it is possible to acquire scalp ringworm from shared pillows, and athlete's foot from shower floors. Body and scalp ringworm may be caught from dogs, cats, and other animals.

Incubation period

is variable, often prolonged.

Infectivity

lasts as long as lesions persist.

Natural history

Scalp ringworm (Tinea capitis)

This starts as a papule and spreads outwards, forming a scaly patch of temporary baldness. The hairs that remain are brittle. There may be progression to a general raised boggy mass (a kerion).

Body ringworm (Tinea corporis)

This is characterized by spreading ring-like lesions with a red, scaly periphery (sometimes with vesicles). As a lesion enlarges the centre often clears to leave normal skin.

Nail ringworm (Tinea unguium)

The nail(s) become discoloured, thick, and brittle. Some white material may accumulate under the nail which itself may eventually disintegrate.

Foot ringworm (Tinea pedis, athlete's foot)

Scaly, itchy lesions develop between the toes (may also occur between fingers). This is more common in older children.

Diagnosis

Except in the easily diagnosed athlete's foot, a skin scraping should be collected. This is done by using a sharp blade to scrape a number of scales from the active edge of the lesion in scalp or body ringworm, or from under the nail. These should be collected on to black (or at least dark) paper and sent to the laboratory for microscopy and culture. Since the characteristic fungal hyphae are usually easily seen under the microscrope, diagnosis can be very rapidly done and reported by telephone.

Management

Scalp ringworm

Although topical treatment can be attempted in many cases this is unsuccessful and a systemic oral anti-fungal agent (griseofulvin) should be used for at least six weeks.

Body ringworm

As for scalp ringworm. Also give a topical anti-fungal preparation (clotrimazole) for two weeks, but impress on the family that the oral medicine is more important.

Nail ringworm

Oral medication (griseofulvin) is essential for up to six months to clear what can be a very persistent infection. Topical medication is ineffective.

Athlete's foot

Unless infection is very extensive, oral anti-fungals are not necessary. Give topical anti-fungal powder or cream (clotrimazole or econazole) and suggest that the feet are kept dry. When many cases of athlete's foot are being reported, check whether standards of hygiene need to be improved in the local school or swimming pool.

Roseola infantum—exanthem subitum

Organism

Probably human herpes virus 6 (HHV6).

Epidemiology

Occurs world-wide as a disease of infancy and early childhood.

Transmission

incubation period, and period of infectivity are all unknown, but unethical experimental studies were performed in the late 1940s in which serum from infected babies was inoculated into healthy infants who developed the illness in nine days.

Natural history

The child has a sudden onset fever with irritability. This lasts 3–5 days with the fever climbing to 40–41°C. The fever suddenly falls and a widespread maculo-papular rash appears (Fig. 2, p. 14).

Diagnosis

Diagnosis is clinical.

Management

Rule out more serious illnesses: see Child with a fever (p. 20) and Child with a rash (p. 11); otherwise symptomatic treatment.

Rubella (German measles)

Notifiable disease
(See Congenital infections: management during pregnancy and the neonatal period)

Organism

Rubella virus.

Epidemiology

Rubella infection in Britain is endemic and epidemics occur every few years (Fig. 5). Infection peaks in the late winter and early spring. In the eighties (when the impact of the immunization programme became apparent) there were 120 cases in the 1983–4 epidemic and 63 cases in the epidemic of 1986–7, which is approximately 5 per 100 000 live births. From 1985 to 1989 there were, on average, 21 cases per year. The number of rubella-associated terminations has fallen considerably, from a maximum

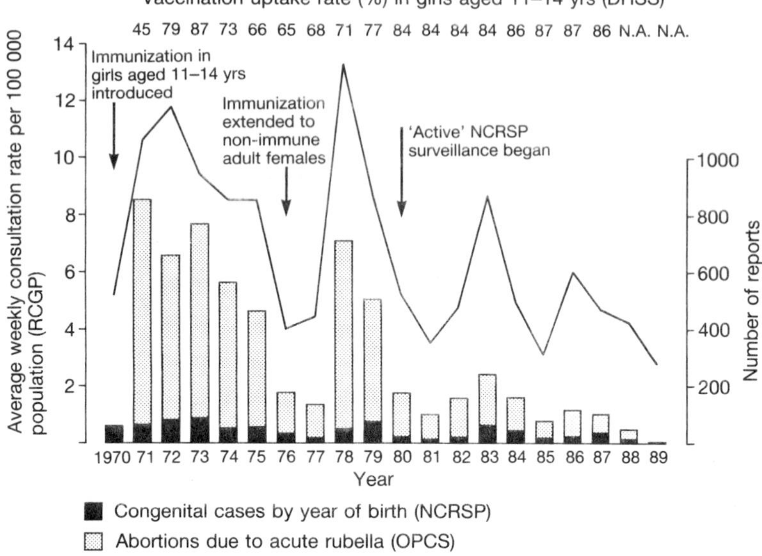

Fig. 5 Incidence of, and immunization against, rubella, England and Wales 1970–89. By courtesy of RCGP, OPCS, NCRSP, and DHSS.

of 830 in 1978 to 44 in 1988. Eighty per cent of cases suffer defects, and pregnancies at particularly high risk are those of Asian mothers who arrived in this country in their teens and who were not reached by the school immunization programme. Reinfection, although rare, has been reported in association with congenital infection.

Transmission

is from nasopharyngeal secretions or urine.

Incubation period

is 14–21 days.

Infectivity

persists from seven days before to seven days after development of the rash in postnatal rubella, while congenitally infected infants may continue to excrete virus for up to a year.

Natural history

Child and adult infection

Prodromal symptoms of infection include a sore throat, cough, and coryza, which may precede the rash by 1–5 days. The rubella rash appears first on the face and spreads to the rest of the body over the next 24 hours (see Fig. 2, p. 14). It is erythematous, and maculo-papular. The lesions on the trunk may coalesce to produce a red blush but those on the limbs remain discrete. The rash appears, spreads and disappears more quickly than that of measles. The rubella rash may be difficult to distinguish from scarlet fever, but in the latter the area around the mouth is spared (circumoral pallor) and the lesions are purple-red rather than pink-red in colour. Enlargement of the posterior auricular and occipital lymph nodes is a characteristic feature of the infection. Arthralgia may occur and encephalitis is a rare complication.

Congenital infection

In those cases where maternal infection was laboratory proven prenatally, no defects have been recorded after the 19th week of pregnancy. Lesions other than deafness are rare after 12 weeks. Congenital rubella is associated with intrauterine growth retardation, thrombocytopenic purpura, congenital heart disease, particularly patent ductus arteriosus and pulmonary arterial or valvar stenosis, mental retardation, microcephaly, cerebral palsy, eye defects, such as cataract and choroidoretinitis, and sensorineural deafness. Multiple defects occur in about one half of infected infants.

Inadvertent immunization just before conception or during the first trimester of pregnancy has not resulted in CRS.

Diagnosis

The clinical diagnosis is difficult to make and may be confused with erythema infectiosum (see p. 54). Suspected rubella during pregnancy, or contact with an infected case, should be investigated using serological tests. Antibodies to the IgG subclass are measured at intervals of 10 days with a radial haemolysis test in acute and convalescent sera, and where there is a fourfold rise confirmation of infection should be made by a measurement of IgM. Many laboratories perform an IgM test initially when rubella infection is suspected during pregnancy. Infection in the neonate can be established either by viral culture of naso-pharyngeal secretions and urine or by serology.

Management

Treatment of rubella in the child or adult is entirely symptomatic. Equally, there is no therapy for congenital infection, but where this is known to have occurred before 18 weeks' gestation termination of pregnancy is recommended. Inadvertent immunization during pregnancy is not an indication for termination. When intra-uterine infection is identified, careful hearing tests, including auditory evoked potentials, should be performed during infancy so that, if required, hearing aids can be fitted at the earliest opportunity. Rubella infection will not recur in subsequent pregnancies.

Confirmed or **suspected** cases of CRS should be reported to the National Congenital Rubella Surveillance Programme as follows:

Professor Catherine Peckham, Dept of Paediatric Epidemiology, The Institute of Child Health, 30 Guilford Street, London WC1N 1EH Tel. 071 242 9789, or Dr Helen Holzel, Dept of Microbiology, Hospital for Sick Children, Great Ormond St, London WC1N 3JH. Tel. 071 405 9200.

Immunization

(See also pp. 172, 184.) Available for girls in secondary school and non-immune adult women. If suspectibility is discovered at antenatal screening, immunization should take place after delivery. History of putative infection is not an excuse for omitting immunization, because a clinical diagnosis of rubella cannot be made with certainty. It is recommended that serology is checked before immunization in girls with arthritis, and vaccine should be avoided where there is active joint disease. Mumps/measles/rubella (MMR) immunization was introduced for pre-school children of both sexes in 1988. Rubella infection is one of the few preventable causes of major handicap in childhood; health premises should display immunization posters and Asian women and other immigrants from less developed countries should be targeted for education in this field. All health workers in contact with pregnant women should ensure that they are themselves immune to infection.

Scabies

Organism

A mite, *Sarcoptes scabiei.*

Epidemiology

Endemic in the UK, this infectious parasite is confined to humans, occurring in adults and children. It is much commoner where standards of hygiene are poor and bathing infrequent.

Transmission

is only by prolonged skin to skin contact.

Incubation period

may be several weeks from first infection to itching; with subsequent infestations the delay is much shorter.

Infectivity

is low but will persist until two courses of treatment have been completed.

Natural history

The female mite burrows into the skin and lays eggs. The patient remains asymptomatic for several weeks until he or she becomes hypersensitive to mite faeces, whereupon intense itchiness develops which is especially troublesome at night. With subsequent infestations the itchiness comes on much earlier as the child's immunity is already primed. There are various signs of the infestation. The burrows of the female may be apparent; tiny wavy lines, sometimes with dark spots inside (the mite or her eggs). Most commonly these are in body folds: the finger webs, wrists, and elbows. When the hypersensitivity reaction has occurred papules, vesicles, or eczematous signs predominate but may be overlaid with the results of scratching. These lesions often occur away from the burrows e.g. on the abdomen and back.

Diagnosis

Essentially this is clinical. The diagnostic signs may be confused by scratching, inappropriate treatment (such as with steroids) and superinfection, and a trial of specific therapy may be useful. If a burrow is seen, mineral oil can be applied to the skin, and a scraping taken and examined microscopically for evidence of mite faecal pellets.

Management

Malathion (Derbac M) or lindane (Quellada) are the treatments of choice. They should be applied to all but the head and neck, allowed to dry, and left for a day without rinsing, and then reapplied after 3 days. Lindane is absorbed through the skin and should be avoided in young children and breastfeeding mothers. To prevent resistance developing, it is recommended that the two drugs are used in rotation. Benzyl benzoate is irritant and crotamiton is ineffective. Children with scabies should not necessarily be excluded from school, though so as to ensure treatment it is sometimes useful to have a local rule of exclusion until the first course of lotion is given.

Staphylococcal infections

Organism

Gram-positive cocci which grow on agar in grape-like clusters. *Staphylococcus aureus* is coagulase positive and *S. epidermidis* is coagulase negative. There are many different strains, many relatively benign, some highly pathogenic.

Epidemiology

S. aureus is carried in the anterior nares of many individuals and *S. epidermidis* can be isolated from the skin of most people.

Transmission

is most commonly person to person via the hands or from the nose.

Incubation period

is 1–10 days for the scalded skin syndrome (a severe generalized skin infection, commonest in the newborn, when it is known as Ritter's disease), but infection frequently arises following prolonged colonization of the mucous membranes of mouth or nose.

Infectivity

is low.

Natural history

Most abscesses and wound infections are caused by *S. aureus*. The umbilicus of the newborn will become colonized by *S. aureus* quickly after birth and, unless the cord is kept clean, omphalitis and then septicaemia may develop. This organism is a cause of furuncles and paronychia in the newborn and, more seriously, of staphylococcal pneumonia, characterized by cavitating lesions and empyema (a collection of pus in the pleural cavity). *S. aureus* is the organism isolated most frequently from the sputum of infants and young children with cystic fibrosis, and is a common cause of cellulitis, osteomyelitis and septic arthritis. Certain toxin-producing strains of *S. aureus* cause food poisoning, scalded skin syndrome, and the toxic shock syndrome (now less common, but associated with tampon use). *S. epidermidis* may colonize indwelling catheters and prostheses and cause disease. Thus *S. epidermidis* may cause meningitis in a child with a ventriculo-peritoneal shunt or septicaemia in patients with central venous catheters.

Diagnosis

By Gram stain, culture, and the coagulase test.

Treatment

Most staphylococci produce penicillinase which inactivates conventional penicillin. Hence the anti-staphylococcal drug of first choice is flucloxacillin, a penicillinase-resistant penicillin. Cephalosporins are alternatives but some broader spectrum drugs, notably ceftazidine are much less effective. When there is multiple drug resistance, vancomycin can be used. Fusidic acid is recommended in combination with another anti-staphylococcal antibiotic in treatment of bone infection or other severe infection. Drainage of free pus should be performed and foreign bodies removed in the presence of infection.

Prevention

In the newborn: handwashing by all attendants is mandatory to prevent epidemics of staphylococcal infection and this will reduce the frequency of other infections. Care of the umbilical stump varies in different centres but antiseptics such as hexachlorophane and chlorhexidine, or topical antibiotics such as polybactrin (a mixture of polymixin B, neomycin, and bacitracin) should be used. Epidemic disease in the newborn nursery is rare but infected infants should be isolated. There is no indication for the treatment of carriers of methicillin-resistant *S. aureus* (MRSA) unless they are long-stay patients or medical staff, in which case topical nasal antibiotics such as 'naseptin' should be used. Many infants and children with cystic fibrosis are treated with oral anti-staphylococcal agents on a long-term basis.

Streptococcal infections

(Excludes *S. pneumoniae*; see p. 94)
Scarlet fever is a notifiable disease

Streptococcus pyogenes or group A streptococcus (beta haemolytic).

Organism

There are at least 75 strains. These are characterized by the 'M' protein in the cell wall.

Epidemiology

Transmission

may occur following inhalation of infected droplets from infected patients or asymptomatic carriers. Impetigo normally develops following direct skin contact. Many of the group A strains are capable of producing rheumatic fever, and glomerulonephritis is associated with a smaller number of strains.

Incubation period

for pharyngitis is 3–5 days, but is longer for impetigo.

Infectivity

from tonsillar or skin colonization may be prolonged.

Natural history

The most common manifestation is tonsillitis or pharyngitis. Scarlet fever patients develop pharyngitis and a characteristic rash produced by an erythrogenic toxin. This rash develops during the first day of fever, is dark-red in colour, and quickly becomes generalized. Lesions are punctate, the size of pinheads, and give the skin a sandpaper-like texture. There is a generalized erythema on the face and forehead, but the area around the mouth is spared (circumoral pallor). Fever peaks on the second day and in untreated infection persists for another 3–4 days. The tonsils are enlarged and covered with exudate. There are characteristic changes to the tongue: for 1–2 days the dorsum is covered in a white fur; the papillae then become red and thickened, protruding through the coat to produce the 'white strawberry tongue'. By the fourth or fifth day the white coat disappears leaving a 'red strawberry tongue'. Petechiae can be seen on the palate during the illness. *Streptococcus pyogenes* is a cause of otitis media. Glomerulonephritis, but not rheumatic fever, may follow skin infections, whereas both conditions may develop after untreated pharyngitis. Cellulitis, septicaemia, endocarditis, and septic arthritis are less usual complications of infection.

Diagnosis

Throat culture is a more reliable method of identification than the rapid antigen identification tests.

Treatment

A throat swab for bacterial culture should be taken from children with acute tonsillitis prior to treatment with antibiotics and it is usually preferable to await the results of culture (available in 24 hours) before starting treatment, particularly as viral tonsillitis caused by adenovirus and Epstein–Barr virus (EBV) cannot be distinguished on clinical grounds. A throat swab should also be taken from children with scarlet fever, although antibiotic treatment can be started once the diagnosis is made. Administration of penicillin for 10 days in the original studies was shown to reduce the risk of rheumatic fever. Penicillin V is the drug of choice, but erythromycin is a satisfactory alternative where there is a definite history of penicillin allergy. There is no indication for the treatment of carriers. Mild impetigo may be treated with topical antibiotics.

Isolation

To prevent epidemics, children should not return to school for at least 24 hours after the start of antimicrobial therapy.

Streptococcus agalactiae or group B streptococcus.

Organism

This is a Gram-positive coccus and is beta haemolytic. (Beta haemolytic describes the clear zone around colonies of bacteria on blood–agar plates.)

Epidemiology

This organism colonizes the genital tract of up to 15 per cent of pregnant women in the UK. Early onset of disease occurs in about one infant for every 100 women colonized, and is more common in the preterm infant.

Transmission

to the newborn occurs *in utero* or during delivery, or may occur from the hands of attendants.

Incubation period

is about three days.

Natural history

Features of **early onset** disease in the newborn include shock, apnoea, and pneumonia. It may be difficult to differentiate such infection from severe idiopathic respiratory distress syndrome. The infection is rapidly progressive. Meningitis is the commonest presentation of **late onset** disease although arthritis, osteomyelitis, and otitis media may occur.

Diagnosis

By Gram stain and culture or antigen detection.

Treatment

Until definite infection with this organism is identified, broad-spectrum treatment should be given. Benzyl penicillin alone is the treatment of choice for both early onset and late onset infection (100 000 u./kg per dose). Recent evidence suggests that ampicillin in large doses to a pregnant carrier mother with prolonged rupture of membranes, or amnionitis (2 g, 4-hourly) may prevent infection in the newborn. There is no indication for the administration of penicillin to well infants found to be colonized after birth.

Tetanus

Notifiable disease

Organism

Clostridium tetani a spore-forming, anaerobic, Gram-positive bacillus.

Epidemiology

Neonatal tetanus is a relatively common cause of death in some less developed countries because of unhygienic birth practices and inadequate care of the umbilical cord stump. In the UK almost all women of childbearing age are immune, so that anti-toxin antibodies are transmitted to the fetus by the trans-placental route, but this is not the case in many developing countries where tetanus immunization is not performed. Neonatal tetanus has been eliminated from the United Kingdom.

Transmission

is by the direct transfer of spores of *C. tetani*, which can be found in soil, and the excreta of animals and humans.

Incubation period

is four days to three weeks.

Natural history

Following contamination of traumatized tissue, burns, or the umbilical stump, spores multiply in anaeobic conditions and produce tetanus toxin which causes powerful muscle contractions, extreme irritability, and death. Case fatality rates in neonates are high.

Diagnosis

This is on clinical grounds. Though infection is more possible in extensive wounds, the wound/site of entry may be trivial. Bacterial culture is positive only in a small proportion of cases.

Treatment

This includes tetanus immune globulin (500–3000 u.), benzyl penicillin for 10–14 days, surgical-wound debridement where indicated, and supportive medical management. Diazepam has proved very beneficial in treating neonatal tetanus. (See also immunization, p. 188.)

Threadworms

Organism

Enterobius vermicularis, a white worm about 2–12 mm long.

Epidemiology

Swallowed ova develop in the small intestine and then colonize the colon. Female worms migrate through the anal orifice, usually at night. Each deposits up to 10 000 ova in the perianal region. There is no secondary host.

Transmission

occurs when scratching begins and eggs accumulate under the finger nails with subsequent spread to other children, parents, and household objects.

Natural history

Infection produces intense perianal itch and irritation, especially at night. This may result in disturbed sleep and screaming episodes on waking.

Diagnosis

Distinctive thread-like worms may be observed in stools. Ova can be collected by pressing adhesive cellophane tape (Sellotape) against the perianal region using a wooden spatula and then looking for eggs microscopically or with a powerful hand magnifier. The best yield occurs in the early morning and parents can be shown how to apply Sellotape which is then brought to the doctor.

Treatment

Piperazine salts or mebendazole as a single dose given to all members of the family. Piperazine should be given on two occasions 14 days apart. Mebendazole should not be given to children under the age of two, and is taken once only. Attention should also be paid to personal hygiene, with a daily bath and hands washed and nails scrubbed before meals.

Thrush (candidiasis)

Organism

Candida albicans, a fungus.

Epidemiology

The normal skin flora includes *Candida* as well as bacteria. Infections are common during infancy, particularly in babies treated with antibiotics, and babies given dummies which become colonized with *Candida* sp.

Transmission

is by direct contact from the birth passages in the newborn infant, or from other sources of infection later. Most infections develop from organisms already present on the skin.

Natural history

Most commonly, this presents either as a white, cheesy deposit in the form of small plaques which may become contiguous on the tongue and inside the cheeks of young babies or as a perianal infection. If severe, the oral infection may interfere with feeding. Nappy rash may also worsen through superinfection. In immunodeficient children, infection is a much more serious problem with widespread severe infection of the skin and mucous membranes with systemic involvement.

Diagnosis

In normal babies the diagnosis is clinical. Because it is a common skin commensal, there is no point in taking samples for culture. The mouth deposit may be confused with milk curds; however, the latter are easily removed with a clean finger while thrush itself requires gentle scraping with a tongue depressor and may leave a bleeding point when removed.

Management

Oral thrush usually responds to nystatin or miconazole and the removal of a dummy if one is being used. Infected nappy rash requires an ointment containing the same agents, perhaps in combination with 1 per cent hydrocortisone.

Treatment of the immunocompromised patient may require both topical therapy and intravenous antifungal agents.

Toxocariasis (visceral larva migrans)

Organism

A nematode; the two main species are *Toxocara canis* and *T. catis*.

Epidemiology

Toxocara canis is a primary infection of dogs which is increasingly being recognized as a hazard to young children (aged 1–4 years), particularly those with pica.

Transmission

occurs when ova from dog faeces are swallowed.

Infectivity

is low. The organism cannot be transmitted from person to person.

Natural history

Symptoms include allergic phenomena such as intermittent fever and asthma. The larvae develop in the small intestine of the child and migrate throughout the body causing allergic phenomena, wheezing, eosinophilia, and splenomegaly. Larvae do not normally mature in the human host. Dead larvae may give rise to endophthalmitis (an eye inflammation) or retinal granulomata and result in loss of vision.

Diagnosis

Eosinophilia and hypergammaglobulinaemia are characteristic. A diagnostic enzyme-linked immunosorbent assay (ELISA) which detects *Toxocara* sp. antibodies is available.

Management

This is with diethylcarbamizine citrate for three weeks. Surgery may be needed to remove granuloma(ta) from the retina.

Prevention

Public education about the danger to young children in allowing public parks to become dogs' lavatories (already the case in most areas). Children's sandpits should be covered to prevent contamination with faeces.

Toxoplasmosis

Organism

Toxoplasma gondii—a protozoan.

Epidemiology

This is a common infection and about half the population of Britain have antibody by middle age. Postnatal acquisition is commonest, but transplacental transmission also occurs in about 30–40 per cent of primary infections in pregnancy, resulting in fetal death or congenital infection.

The incidence of toxoplasmosis during pregnancy in the west of England and South Wales is about 2:1000, but the incidence of congenital infection is unknown, because the disease is difficult to diagnose, and because the majority of symptomatic cases present with choroidoretinitis which may not become apparent until late childhood. Each year 100–300 cases of choroidoretinitis in patients with toxoplasma antibodies are reported, but it is not known how many of these are caused by toxoplasmosis. Preliminary reports to the BPSU suggest that there are 10–20 babies delivered each year in the UK who show signs of toxoplasmosis during early infancy.

In France, where antenatal sera have been tested for toxoplasma infection for many years, about 7 per cent of maternal infections lead to symptomatic infection during infancy and childhood.

Transmission

is poorly understood but is probably by two principal routes: consumption of undercooked meat containing the tissue cyst of *T. gondii*, and direct contact with soil contaminated with the oocyst stage of the organism's life cycle which is shed by domestic cats during acute infection. There is some evidence for transmission via unpasteurized milk (particularly from goats) and via water.

Incubation period

depends on the infecting dose and is probably about 10–14 days.

Period of infectivity

Infection is not transmitted from one individual to another.

Natural history

Postnatal infection

90 per cent of patients are asymptomatic and the remainder develop a glandular fever-like or non-specific febrile illness associated with lymphadenopathy. Occasional severe systemic invasive infection is more likely in the immunocompromised patient but can occur in the immunocompetent. Complete recovery is usual, but tissue cysts and antibody persist for life. Reactivated cysts may lead to recurrent disease if the host becomes immunocompromised.

Congenital infection

A small proportion of infected infants present with the classic triad of hydrocephalus, choroidoretinitis, and intracranial calcification. Other babies may appear normal but develop choroidoretinitis.

Diagnosis

Infection in pregnancy

By serology—several specific enzyme linked immuno-assay (ELISA) IgM assays are available which indicate infection over the previous 6 months. The toxoplasma dye test and a number of other IgG tests are also in use. When there is serological evidence of maternal infection, fetal blood sampling is recommended for both serology and culture of *T. gondii*.

Congenital infection

This can be detected by serology on cord blood and also by culture. If there is a strong clinical suspicion of infection, then serology should be performed for the first year at 3-monthly intervals, as antibodies may be slow to rise.

Management

Infection in pregnancy

Unfortunately there have been no control trials of treatment of toxoplasmosis during pregnancy and infancy. It is recommended that maternal infection is treated with spiramycin until the results of fetal serology are known. If serology is positive then pyrimethamine, sulphadiazine, and folinic acid should be given daily for 3 weeks and then alternated with spiramycin until delivery. If fetal blood sampling is not possible then spiramycin alone can be given. Infection during the first trimester carries a significant risk of fetal damage. When this has been confirmed by fetal serology, termination of pregnancy is a reasonable option. To avoid termination of normal fetuses, this procedure should not be performed unless fetal infection has been confirmed.

Treatment of the newborn

If there is no evidence of infection (by serology and culture), either *in utero* or at birth, then spiramycin can be given until 6 months, providing serology remains negative. When there has been fetal infection (IgM antibodies in fetal blood sample, or cord blood) then alternating courses of pyrimethamine and sulphonamide and spiramycin should be given in the first year of life.

Any infant with suspected or proven infection should be assessed by an ophthalmologist, and undergo ultrasound and CT scan of the brain to look for calcification.

Prevention

This is directed at preventing acquisition in pregnancy and can be summarized: 'Wash your hands thoroughly before eating or touching your face (particularly in the company of cats) and cook your meat thoroughly (brown right through).' The desirability of screening for infection during pregnancy is being considered at present.

Tuberculosis (TB)

Notifiable disease

Organism

Mycobacterium tuberculosis. Also referred to as an acid fast bacillus (AFB) (see Diagnosis). Atypical (non-tuberculous) mycobacterium causes milder disease.

Epidemiology

Incidence and mortality are now low in the UK, having fallen as living standards have risen. Estimates of incidence taken from a survey of cases in 1983 in different racial groups were as follows: white 2.6/100 000, Indian 34/100 000, Pakistani/ Bangladeshi 54/100 000. Second-generation immigrants are at lower risk and rates in West Indian children are not demonstrably higher than in white children. Certain groups of children are at high risk of infection: those in close contact with active (especially open pulmonary) TB; children recently coming from less developed countries; children in British Asian and African families and those with AIDS.

Transmission

is by airborne spread from sputum of infected contacts with open pulmonary TB.

Incubation period

from infection to primary lesion is 1–3 months.

Infectivity

is low. Usually this requires prolonged, close contact (e.g. sharing living accommodation). Infection through brief contact is extremely rare. Children are, on the whole, much less infectious than adults. When a case occurs in a school it is more important to look for the infecting adult, and the child should be isolated only if a sputum smear is positive. Tuberculosis affecting organs other than the lungs is not a risk to others. More commonly the problem arises as to how long to keep parents with 'open' TB away from their children. In this situation BCG (Bacillus Calmette–Guerin vaccine) should be given to the child and the parent(s) regarded as non-infectious following a few weeks of treatment, this being checked by smear testing of sputum. Where parent–child separation is undesirable, e.g. a mother with her newborn, treatment may be commenced in the asymptomatic baby (see p. 35).

Natural history

The organism almost always enters via the respiratory tract and primary infection occurs in the lung (primary focus, Ghon complex). Usually there is complete resolution or a small area of calcification following some localized inflammation (pneumonitis) and enlarged lymph nodes (hilar lymphadenopathy).

This process commonly goes undetected as the child seems well. Children may, however, become unwell if the infection proceeds, although mild disease can be undistinguishable from a simple respiratory infection with fever. Unless a tuberculous cause is suspected (e.g. known contact) the diagnosis may be missed. In a small number of children, there is direct spread to the lungs (bronchopneumonia), systemic spread to the lungs and other organs (miliary TB), or localization of infection following systemic spread to the meninges, bone, or kidneys. If infection is acquired by drinking infected (unpasteurized) milk abroad, cervical lymph node disease or gastrointestinal TB occurs. Malnourished children and those who have not had BCG are more likely to progress to severe disease.

Diagnosis

When tuberculosis is suspected, the child should be referred to a paediatrician who is likely to consult a chest physician or infectious disease specialist once the diagnosis has been made. Investigations should include a CXR and a tuberculin skin test: either a

Heaf test (see p. 193) or a Mantoux test, in which 0.1 ml of 1 u. 1000 tuberculin, 100 u./ml is injected intradermally. The Mantoux test is positive when the diameter of the area of induration is more than 6 mm 48–72 h after the test has been performed. Weaker reactions may be due to prior BCG, infection with atypical (non-tuberculous) mycobacterium, or early disease.

A definitive diagnosis can be made by identification of acid fast bacilli, using the Ziehl–Nielsen stain; these may be seen on gastric washings, sputum, pleural or cerebrospinal fluid, urine, or other body fluids. These specimens should be cultured but the tubercle bacillus grows slowly and a positive result may not be obtained for up to six weeks. Further identification of infection may be made by histological examination; giant cells and tubercle bacilli may be seen in biopsy specimens from infected children.

Tuberculous meningitis is diagnosed following examination of cerebrospinal fluid (CSF). Most commonly there is a lymphocytosis, though early on neutrophils can predominate or the specimen may occasionally be cell-free; protein concentration is usually high and glucose low (under 50 per cent of value in blood taken simultaneously). If TB meningitis is suspected, the laboratory must be told so that the special stains and culture can be performed. The CSF should always be cultured so that the sensitivity of the organisms can be determined. It may sometimes be difficult to make the diagnosis from CSF examination and a tuberculin test should be performed immediately.

Management

This should be performed jointly by a paediatrician and chest physician or infectious disease specialist.

The newborn infant

There is rarely a need for separation of the mother with TB from her infant; breast feeding is not contraindicated during treatment with antituberculous drugs. The alternative forms of management in well babies are dependent on the disease status of the mother, as follows.

Mother with positive tuberculin test and no evidence of active disease

(assuming the mother has not been immunized previously): BCG can be given either at birth or within the first week of life.

Mother with positive tuberculin test and undergoing treatment for primary tuberculosis

Isoniazid should be given for six months to one year and isoniazid-resistant BCG administered after birth. The infant should be separated from the mother **only** while she is considered infectious (usually 2–4 weeks after the start of treatment).

Mother with haematogenous TB, such as miliary TB, TB meningitis

Following investigation of the infant to exclude congenital TB, give isoniazid for 6–12 months and isoniazid-resistant BCG after birth.

Infant with congenital TB

Treat with isoniazid and rifampicin for a minimum of nine months.

BCG should not be given to any baby delivered to an HIV-positive mother because of the risk of 'BCG osis'. BCG does not produce immunity to TB in all infants and for this reason some physicians use chemotherapy alone in the newborn.

Later infancy and childhood

When a child is found to have a positive tuberculin skin test and there is no previous history of BCG immunization or evidence of active disease, isoniazid should be given for 12 months.

Children with pulmonary TB are best treated with a nine-month regimen; isoniazid and rifampicin are the drugs of choice. When it is thought that drug resistance is a possibility (and this is uncommon), a third drug should be added for the first two months of treatment: ethambutol, pyrazinamide, or streptomycin can be used. Ethambutol may cause an optic neuritis, which resolves if the drug is stopped in the early stages. Regular visual tests have to be performed, but interpretation may be difficult in the younger child so the drug should not be used in children under the age of six. Streptomycin causes vestibular and cochlear damage, the risk increasing with higher cumulative doses, so it should not be used for more than two months. Pyrazinamide may cause hepatitis; the preparation available in the UK is not licensed for use in children but is acceptable and has a place in the treatment of tuberculous meningitis (see below).

Miliary TB and tuberculous meningitis, as well as TB in other extra-pulmonary sites, should be treated with a minimum of three drugs: ethambutol, or pyrazinamide, or streptomycin given for the first two months should be combined with isoniazid and rifampicin, which should be given for a minimum of 18 months. Pyrazinamide reaches therapeutic concentrations in the cerebrospinal fluid and is used in both the UK and USA for children with tuberculous meningitis. There is no place for intra-thecal treatment in this condition.

Typhoid fever

Notifiable disease

Organism

Salmonella typhi, a bacterium.

Epidemiology

There are between 50 and 60 notifications of typhoid fever in children each year in England and Wales; most disease is acquired overseas, chiefly in the Indian subcontinent.

Transmission

is by contaminated food or water through the faecal–oral route.

Incubation period

depends on the size of the infecting dose. The usual range is 1 3 weeks.

Infectivity

Untreated cases may excrete the organism indefinitely after recovery, and asymptomatic carriers can be an important source of infection for long periods.

Natural history

The disease is usually mild in infants and more serious in older children and adults. Severe cases have sustained fever of insidious onset with malaise. Illness is associated with either diarrhoea or constipation and cough. Physical signs include hepatomegaly, splenomegaly, and rose-red spots on the trunk.

Diagnosis

This is primarily by blood cultures, but the organism can sometimes be cultured from stools or urine. Serological tests do not have a place in diagnosis.

Management

If this disease is suspected, rapid referral to a paediatrician is mandatory. Treatment will include intravenous fluids and chloramphenicol (see Gastroenteritis, p. 56). The Medical Officer of Environmental Health needs to be involved urgently for contact tracing.

Varicella (see chickenpox).

Warts and verrucae

Organism

The human papilloma virus (HPV) or warts virus, of which there are a number of sub-types. Certain sub-types of HPV are associated with genital warts.

Epidemiology

Occurs world-wide in adults and children.

Transmission

is by direct contact, but with low infectivity. There is no good evidence that verrucae can be acquired from swimming-pool floors. The warts virus can be transmitted sexually.

Incubation period

has a large range from one month to two years.

Infectivity

may last as long as lesions persist.

Natural history

The appearance of warts is well known. It is less frequently appreciated that verrucae are warts occurring on the feet (plantar warts). The latter may be tender or associated with a 'pricking' sensation. Warts elsewhere are usually painless. The appearance varies with site: on the hands, face, and knees warts tend to be smooth and flat; in the genital and peri-anal regions they are larger, filiform, and fast-growing (condyloma acuminata); verrucae on the feet have the appearance of warts growing inwards.

Diagnosis

This is clinical. DNA analysis may be used to type a genital wart in cases of suspected sexual abuse.

Management

Warts on the hands and feet are difficult to treat, and topical preparations are not always effective. For symptomatic warts on the feet a pumice stone can be used to pare off the surface layer; application of dry ice can be considered. Most warts resolve spontaneously and do not require treatment.

Exceptions are genital warts, which may be acquired following sexual abuse. (Some genital sub-types of HPV may be associated with cervical carcinoma.) Children with genital warts should be referred to a paediatrician. There is no need to exclude children with verrucae from swimming or to force them to wear special socks.

Whooping cough (pertussis)

Notifiable disease

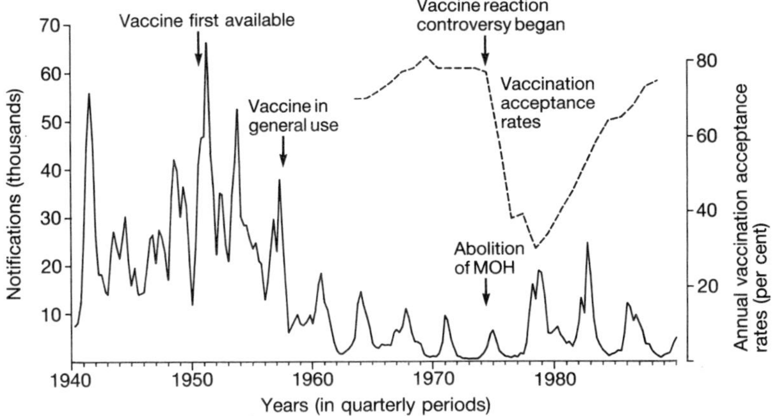

Fig. 6 Quarterly notifications of whooping cough, England and Wales 1940–89. By courtesy of CDSC. Prepared from material provided by OPCS and DHSS.

Organism

Bordetella pertussis, a Gram-negative bacterium.

Epidemiology

Whooping cough remains a common childhood disease in the UK. Epidemics occur at four-year intervals with peak incidence during the winter months. The last was in 1985–6; the next will be in 1989–90. When immunization rates were relatively high, epidemics were only moderate in size. However, following loss of public and professional confidence in the vaccine, in 1974 immunization coverage declined to 30 per cent and the scale of epidemics was greatly magnified (Fig. 6). Notified mortality from pertussis is relatively low (64 deaths from 1976 to 1985); however, these figures may be an under-estimate because it is possible the disease may go undiagnosed in some infant respiratory and 'cot deaths' where the presentation is without a characteristic cough and whoop.

Transmission

is by droplet spread or direct contact with discharge from the nose and mouth (including soiled handkerchiefs). Older children and adults may also have the disease in an unrecognized form and transmit it to young children.

Incubation period
is 7–10 days.

Infectivity
is highest in the catarrhal stage, but can be prolonged for up to a month after the start of the cough unless an appropriate antibiotic is given. When this is done, a child or adult becomes non-infectious in about five days (though the cough itself persists).

Natural history

Initially the child has a runny nose (catarrhal phase) followed in about two days by a cough which gradually becomes paroxysmal. During the bouts of coughing the baby or child may become red or blue/black in the face from hypoxia. One Asian word for the disease means 'the black cough'. When the bout stops, the child catches his or her breath, inspires in a rush, and causes the characteristic 'whoop'. Vomiting is common, and in young infants feeding may become impossible. Terminal apnoea is a significant risk in young babies following loss of consciousness with hypoxia. The cough gradually subsides, but bouts may persist for a number of months. A Chinese pictogram for pertussis can be interpreted as 'the illness of a hundred days'. Complications include pneumonia, encephalitis, convulsions, and cerebral damage.

Diagnosis

In a classical case this may be made on clinical signs as, once heard, the 'whoop' is rarely forgotten. However, it is important to confirm the diagnosis in all cases, particularly where the presentation is atypical, because other organisms (adenoviruses and *Bordetella parapertussis*) can produce similar illnesses. A diagnosis cannot be made using a throat swab. Instead a per-nasal swab (a swab on a four-inch flexible metal wand) should be inserted through the nose to take a sample from the back of the nasopharynx. This is unpleasant for the child and will often precipitate a bout of coughing. The swab is then placed in Stuart's medium and sent for culture or immunofluorescence. Because these swabs are positive in only about half the cases during the catarrhal stage of the illness, a negative result does not refute the clinical diagnosis. A substantial lymphocytosis is common in the early stages, but not diagnostic.

Management

Erythromycin given early in the catarrhal stage may shorten the illness. This antibiotic is recommended for all children with pertussis to render them non-infectious, which takes about five days. This is particularly important when a child develops pertussis and there is a young infant in the household. It is quite acceptable in these situations to give erythromycin to the infant (even if asymptomatic) if the primary immunization course has not been completed.

The disease is hardest to manage in young babies where the paroxysms of coughing can be extremely frightening for the parents. Phenobarbitone is useful in reducing the frequency and severity of coughing paroxysms. To avoid vomiting, small, frequent feeds are advisable. Managing a baby at home can be both exhausting and stressful, and admission is often necessary for social reasons. When the child is having cyanotic attacks, admission is indicated for medical reasons because of the danger of terminal apnoea. In hospital the infant should be nursed in a cubicle until non-infectious. Tube feeding is often required. High levels of nurse staffing are needed because of the frequent attention these infants require when having coughing bouts. Microphone systems and apnoea alarms may be required to alert staff to an episode.

In the recovery phase the older child may be allowed to return to school. It will be necessary to explain to the teachers that despite its cough the child is not a risk to others. When a case or epidemic occurs strenuous efforts should be made to ensure that all contacts are up to date with their immunizations.

Yellow fever

Notifiable disease

Organism

An arborvirus.

Epidemiology

Yellow fever occurs in two endemic zones in Central Africa and northern South America with a natural reservoir in forest monkeys; however, cases occur in both urban and rural settings with a relatively high mortality. The disease is almost unheard of in the UK, but British travellers to endemic zones are at risk.

Transmission

is by mosquito, either between monkey and man or man to man.

Incubation period

is 3–6 days.

Natural history

A disease of varying severity which in severe forms manifests as sudden onset fever, malaise proceeding to jaundice, haemorrhagic symptoms, and death.

Diagnosis

This is by isolation of the virus or serological testing.

The collection of specimens for the diagnosis of infection

General principles

If in doubt whether to take a sample, what to take, or how to send it, the laboratory should be consulted first. As a rule, specimens should be collected only when results may affect management, or in the investigation of outbreaks of infection. The diagnostic tests for individual diseases are given in Table 12. In writing the request card remember that this is usually all the information that the laboratory has to go on. Therefore give details of:

the child's name and date of birth (not just his or her age);
the doctor's name, address, and telephone number;
the illness, its date of onset, and main clinical features;
treatment (particularly anti-microbials) and its duration;
relevant infectious disease contacts;
any recent foreign travel;
details (with dates) of previous samples.

Equipment

A clinic or practice will need the following:

swabs, including the per-nasal variety (see p. 137);
transport medium: Stuart's, chlamydial, and viral;
universal containers and 'dip slides' (if delay is anticipated);
faeces containers;
blood-taking equipment suitable for children ('butterflies', small-gauge hypodermic needles);
blood bottles suitable for small samples.

Collection—transport—storage

Blood

Most serological tests can be achieved with 2–5 ml, but it may be necessary to check with the laboratory the minimum amount required. An initial explanation that the patient is a child will often reduce the volume asked for. The sample can usually be stored at 4°C overnight. (Blood cultures are an exception, but these are rarely taken outside hospital.) Collection of blood from young children is not easy. Butterfly needles (green or blue) are useful because 'flashback' occurs once the needle enters the vein, and they tolerate greater movement of the child than ordinary needles before becoming dislodged. **Never collect blood from a vessel in the groin** and refer to an experienced children's doctor if sampling is difficult.

Table 12 Diagnostic tests for individual diseases

	Disease	Specimen	Method of diagnosis
★	AIDS/HIV	Blood	Antibody test (Antigen test also done but expensive) Label 'High Risk' (red star). In acquired infection, antibodies may not be present for 3 months or more, although antigen can sometimes be detected earlier. Interpretation of results in children prior to 15 months is problematic because of antibody from the mother.
	Chickenpox/ herpes zoster	Vesicle swab	Culture, serology, and electron microscopy of vesicle fluid available
△	Chlamydia	Neonates: eye swab or nasopharyngeal aspirate	Chlamydia transport-medium or special microscope slide.
		Older children: other swabs	Chlamydia transport-medium. Where sexual abuse suspected tissue culture must be performed (p. 32)
★ △	Cholera	Stool/rectal swab	Diagnosis is by microscopy and culture; serology also available
	Congenital cytomegalovirus	Urine Throat swab	Send promptly to lab.; serology inconclusive.
△	Diphtheria	Throat swab	**If suspected consult immediately.** If *C. diphtheriae* found, lab. will test whether a toxin-producing strain

Table 12 *continued*

Disease	Specimen	Method of diagnosis
Gastrointestinal infections:		
△ *Campylobacter*	Stool	Culture.
Cryptosporidium	Stool	Microscopy for cysts.
E. coli	Stool	Culture.
Giardia	Stool	Microscopy for cysts. Duodenal aspirate can be done in hospital.
Rotavirus	Stool	ELISA or electron microscopy.
△ *Salmonella*	Stool (not rectal swab)	Two specimens on separate days preferable for bacterial culture
△ *Shigella*	Stool	Bacterial culture.
Glandular fever or infectious mononucleosis	Blood	Full blood count and film will show lymphocytosis; serology using Bunnell or monospot test may not be positive for a month.
Haemophilus influenzae	Swab	Bacterial culture.
★ △ Gonorrhoea	Neonates: eye swab Older children: swabs; put in medium to prevent drying.	See the child with sexually transmitted disease (p. 31).
△ Hepatitis A	± serum	Clinical diagnosis sufficient in most cases; antibody tests are available but rarely justified.
△ △ Hepatitis B	Blood	Test for surface antigen. Specimens must be marked 'High Risk' (red star).

Table cont. on next page

Table 12 *continued*

	Disease	Specimen	Method of diagnosis
★	Herpes simplex	—	Clinical diagnosis sufficient. Tissue culture is available but serology is not useful.
	Influenza	—	Clinical diagnosis sufficient. Viral culture of secretions collected on a nose or throat swab may occasionally be indicated.
★ △	Malaria	Blood	Examination of thick film or smear by an experienced person. This is an urgent investigation. Crucial to specify country of travel and anti-malarials taken.
△	Measles	Blood	Clinical diagnosis. Serology is available.
★ △	Meningococcal disease	Blood Cerebrospinal fluid (CSF)	Microscopy of CSF; bacterial culture; if suspected, for immediate referral (see p. 88).
	Molluscum contagiosum	—	Clinical diagnosis
△	Mumps	—	Viral isolation and serology available but normally unnecessary as clinical diagnosis straightforward.
	Pneumococcus	Swab	Bacterial culture.
★ △	Polio	—	Urgent referral where suspected.
	Respiratory syncytial virus	Nasopharyngeal aspirate	Immunofluorescence or viral culture.

Table 12 *continued*

	Disease	Specimen	Method of diagnosis
	Rubella	Blood (adult) Viral swab (newborn)	Serology in adult; culture in newborn
	Staphylococcus aureus	Swab	Bacterial culture.
	Streptococcal disease	Swab Serology	Laboratories will 'type' looking for group A haemolytic forms; antistreptolysin O titre useful in care of rheumatic fever and acute glomerulonephritis.
★	Tetanus	—	Urgent referral where suspected.
	Thrush	—	Clinical diagnosis.
	Tinea	Skin scrapings	Culture.
★ △	Tuberculosis	Sputum Urine	Refer immediately when child is ill; if child is well perform Heaf test.
★ △	Typhoid	Stool Blood culture	Culture for *S. typhi.*
	Warts	—	Clinical diagnosis; DNA analysis where thought to result from sexual abuse.
	Whooping cough	Per-nasal swab	Special swab on flexible wand inserted into the nasopharynx through the nose; put into Stuart's medium.
★	Yellow fever	—	Urgent referral if suspected.

★ Prior consultation of laboratory/paediatrician essential.
△ Contact the Medical Officer of Environmental Health who will initiate relevant contact-tracing and other preventive activities.

Only routinely available tests are noted. Special tests are available for many of the diseases but will usually require consultation. Many of the infections listed are discussed in greater detail in the Diseases section.

Skin scrapings

(Tinea) Collect for fungal hyphae by scraping with a blade from the edge of a lesion on to black paper (so that the white scrapings can be found), fold this carefully, put it in a universal container and send, requesting microscopy and culture.

Stool specimens

Where microscopy is required it is better to send fresh specimens. Optimal practice is to get samples for bacterial culture and viral identification to the laboratory the same day; if stored overnight this must be in a refrigerator at 4°C. On the request form it is particularly important to say whether a search for ova, cysts, and parasites is needed, and/or a culture, and whether the child has been anywhere abroad.

Swabs

Always put these into appropriate transport media. Apart from chlamydia and viruses (needing special media) all swabs can go in Stuart's medium. Swabs from skin lesions need to be from an exudate or a damp area. This may mean lifting scabs or expressing pus/vesicular fluid. Throat swabs must be from the tonsils or any other area where an exudate or lesions are seen. Per-nasal swabs for detection of *Bordetella pertussis* require a special technique (see p. 137). Vaginal swabs should be collected from the vestibular fossa by gently drawing apart the labia minora. Rectal swabs need to be inserted just inside the anus. Specimens should, whenever possible, reach the lab within four hours. When overnight storage is unavoidable, keep them at 4°C; they must not be frozen.

Urine

In older children collect mid-stream samples using the same technique as for adults. In infants and younger children a clean catch specimen is best. This involves waiting with the partially naked child until he or she 'pees'. Then a sterile container is placed in the stream of urine. The technique demands infinite patience but it is far less susceptible to contamination than the stick-on urine bags. Drinks of orange and running taps help to speed up the process. Often it is most conveniently done in the clinic or ward by the parents. If a urine bag is used the perineum should be cleaned gently with water (not antiseptic) before this is applied. It is best to leave it exposed to view so that urine is removed immediately it is seen. Supra-pubic aspiration of urine with a needle and syringe is sometimes necessary but should be done in hospital.

Immunization

General introduction

Artificial immunity is achieved in two ways, active and passive. Active immunity is long lasting and is achieved with injected and oral vaccines. Passive immunity is short lived and comes from the injection of immunoglobulins. This section describes the principal vaccines and immunoglobulins available in the UK, their uses, and handling.

Vaccines are customarily divided into two groups: those that are live but attenuated and those that have been inactivated.

Live vaccines

BCG
Measles
Measles/mumps/rubella (MMR)
Mumps
Polio (oral form, OPV)
Rubella
Yellow fever

These are highly effective: by inducing a slight infection they give many years of protection, often from a single dose. Yet, apart occasionally from oral polio, the infection is not communicable to others.

Inactivated vaccines

Cholera
Diphtheria*
Hepatitis B
Influenza
Pertussis
Pneumococcus
Polio (injectable, IPV)
Rabies
Tetanus*
Typhoid

(*The vaccines for diphtheria and tetanus are preparations from the bacterial exotoxins rather than the bacteria organism itself.

They are sometimes referred to as toxoid vaccines.) A single dose of inactivated vaccine tends to be less effective than a live preparation equivalent (notably so for typhoid and cholera) and multiple doses are usually needed to give long-term protection.

Increasingly vaccines employ sub-units of the pathogenic organism to promote a protective effect, and in the future we can anticipate entirely engineered synthetic vaccines. Despite this diversity, all vaccines work on the same principle: that by simulating response to a pathogen they induce active immunity. All the vaccines described below have been through a rigorous testing process before being licensed for use. However, there is no such thing as a perfect vaccine. Each has its own degree of effectiveness, indications, contraindications, and reactions, and immunizers must be aware of these or know where to find out details.

For each vaccine there is an immunization strategy. These fall into two broad types. Firstly, of protecting the susceptibles: this means providing immunity to individual children or adults at risk from the disease. This may be all individuals (eg for tetanus) or only a limited number (eg for pneumococcal disease). Secondly, that of reducing the circulation of disease-producing organisms. This works on a mass basis whereby if enough adults and children are vaccinated (high 'herd immunity'), and humans are the only host for a disease, then the organism may eventually die out, assuming there is no carrier state; or at least there will be little of the disease in circulation. Oral polio has worked in this way and the same could be achieved for measles and rubella.

Contraindications

There are circumstances when vaccines must not be given, both general and specific.

General contraindications

Acute febrile illness

A temperature over 37.5°C (38°C rectally). If a child has an acute febrile illness, the immunization must not be given because, if the condition worsens, diagnostic difficulties will arise as to whether the deterioration is due to the immunization or the illness. Since immunization is almost always an elective procedure, it is sensible to delay this until the child is well on the way to recovery.

Specific contraindications

The following contraindications and special considerations apply for all **live vaccines** (see list, p. 143).

Antibiotic sensitivity

All live vaccines contain minute traces of antibiotics necessary in their preparation, most commonly neomycin and polymixin. Extremely rarely, individuals have an anaphylactic reaction to a specific antibiotic and they should not receive a vaccine with the antibiotic concerned. However, most sensitivity to neomycin and polymixin is a mild contact-dermatitis or delayed hypersensitivity which are **not** contraindications.

Pregnancy

None of the vaccines in current use have been shown to cause fetal malformations. However, unless there are compelling reasons (e.g. an unprotected woman about to go to a yellow fever zone or endemic polio area) it seems wise to avoid immunization in the first four months of pregnancy. **It should be specifically noted that rubella immunization in early pregnancy is no longer a reason for advising termination** (see p. 186).

Giving multiple live vaccines

Two or more live vaccines may be given simultaneously (e.g. MMR). However, on theoretical grounds once one has been given three weeks should elapse before the next live vaccine is administered (see also BCG, p. 190).

Immunodeficient children

A live vaccine may overwhelm a child who is seriously immunodepressed and live vaccines should not be given to such children. This does not apply to the child with HIV infection who can be given the oral polio vaccine and MMR (see p. 217).

Inactivated vaccines

(See p. 143 for list.) Attention must be paid to the contraindications for each vaccine. The issues of antibiotic sensitivity, pregnancy, and multiple vaccine administration are of less practical significance than for live vaccines. Inactivated vaccines can be given to all immunodeficient individuals, although they may not be very affective in this group.

Individual specific contraindications and children with problem histories

Individual vaccines carry a number of specific contraindications and these are detailed below under each vaccine. When these apply, a child must not be immunized. (An example is pertussis vaccine when there has been a prior severe reaction.) There are also circumstances (previously referred to as special considerations) where immunization is perhaps thought to be associated with a somewhat increased risk. These are referred to as children with problem histories and detailed in the notes at the end of each immunization section. An example would be immunizing a child with a convulsive tendency with MMR vaccine. Any additional risk must always be weighed against the danger associated with leaving the child unprotected. Each child needs individual assessment but, on balance, most children with problem histories should be immunized. In the example given a British child with febrile convulsions is 8–10 times more likely to suffer a further fit because of measles than from the vaccine.

Adsorbed and plain killed vaccines

The three components of the Triple vaccine (diphtheria/tetanus/pertussis) are available in plain form or adsorbed in an aluminium hydroxide suspension both in the individual (monovalent) and combined preparations. The one exception is monovalent pertussis which is available only in a plain form. Sometimes doctors use the plain form preparations where there have been local reactions to previous injections, as these seem to occur less frequently with the plain preparations. However, this is rarely an issue in children and, as a rule, the adsorbed should be used as it gives somewhat better protection.

Mythical contraindications

Both primary care and hospital practice are permeated with mythical reasons for children being denied protection. Unfortunately, many of these have been communicated to the public. The

following conditions are **not** reasons for a child being denied protection through immunization.
The child (or any family member):
suffering from eczema, asthma, or hay fever;
receiving antibiotics;
receiving low-dose or topical steroids;
having a history of neonatal jaundice;
a baby being under a certain weight;
having a prior history of pertussis, measles, or rubella except for proven infection;
suffering from chestiness or snuffles;
suffering from 'underdevelopment';
having been born prematurely;
suffering from a stable neurological condition;
suffering from syndromes such as Down's or Turner's. Likewise, there is no contraindication to immunization when a child's mother is pregnant or breastfeeding.

When a child is believed to have a contraindication to any immunization this must not be accepted on verbal basis alone. No indicated immunization must be denied to a child without careful verification by consulting this volume or the DOH *Immunization against infectious disease*. Where doubt remains specialist advice must be sought rather than omitting the immunization. Each Health District (Health Board in Scotland) has an individual designated as responsible for immunization and able to give an expert opinion.

Vaccine handling

When vaccines are received from the pharmacy, chemist, or any other source they should be placed immediately in the main body of the refrigerator, not in the door section (where the temperature will rise on opening) or the freezing compartment. All vaccines must be protected from light. Maximum and minimum thermometers are necessary for vaccine fridges and these should be checked regularly.

Transport of vaccines and use in satellite clinics

Vaccines allowed to warm up will not work

In many circumstances vaccines have to be transported by staff to peripheral centres before their use. When this happens they must be kept at their correct cold-storage temperature while in transit and at the peripheral centre. This is called a 'cold chain'.

Guidelines for maintaining a successful cold chain are:

1. Rigid cool boxes with well-fitting lids and two ice ('freezer') packs should be used for transport. Soft bags are not acceptable.
2. Excessive amounts of vaccine should not be taken out in cool boxes, and what is taken must be loaded into the cool box as close to the departure time as possible, so as to minimize the time out of the fridge.
3. Vaccines should be kept in the cool box with the ice packs throughout the session. The lid must be kept on the box as much as possible.
4. Unused vaccine should be returned to the main fridge as soon as practicable after the session is over.
5. Where repeated exposure of vaccines to higher temperatures has been unavoidable, they should be dated and used within two weeks.

Disposal

At the end of the session any prepared or opened vaccine must be destroyed. The label needs to be defaced with a ballpoint pen and the ampoules put into a 'burn bin'. Alternatively vaccines can be returned to a pharmacy, in which case they should be transported in a sealed bag within a pharmacy box. Burn bins should not be stored in satellite clinics but returned to the main centre.

Disposal of BCG vaccine and tuberculin PPD

Any remaining vaccine must be drawn into a syringe and placed in a burn bin for return to the health centre and incineration. Alternatively, it can be returned in a sealed box within a pharmacy box. Expired vaccines should also be placed in a burn bin or in a sealed bag in a locked box for return to the pharmacy. **Under no circumstances should vaccines, syringes, needles, or empty ampoules be disposed of in any way in the health centre/**

Table 13 Required storage conditions for vaccines

Tetanus Diphtheria Dip./Tet. Dip./Tet./pertussis Hepatitis B Pertussis Adult diphtheria Typhoid	2–8°C **Do not freeze**	Refrigerator, not freezing compartment
MMR Measles Rubella BCG	2–8°C **Do not freeze**	Dried MMR, measles, and rubella have a shelf-life of 2 yr at 2–8°C, but only 10 weeks at room temperature. BCG 1–2 yr at 2–8°C, but only one month at room temperature. All should be used within 8 h of reconstitution
Oral polio	2–6°C (Smith, Kline, and French) 0–4°C (Wellcome)	Refrigerator, not freezing compartment. Occasional exposure up to 25°C is permissible **but each exposure must not exceed 2 h.** (Oral polio vaccine may be frozen; bulk supplies are stored at −20°C)
Tuberculin PPD	2–8°C **Do not freeze**	Discard one hour after opening

clinic except by incineration in burn bins. They must not be put into ordinary waste bags and bins.

Accidental spillage of vaccine

Wash the contaminated surface with a suitable disinfectant, such as sodium hypochlorite 0.3–0.4 per cent (Chlorasol).

Preparing for immunization, medical prescriptions, nurse immunizing, and parental consent

At the start of an immunization session, the vaccines, the equipment for vaccination, and the equipment and drugs for treatment of anaphylaxis must all be checked (see also p. 153).

Any child presenting for immunization has to be indiviually assessed by the nurse or doctor for: the indicated immunization; any contraindications; the child's fitness for immunization that day. If a nurse is immunizing and there is any doubt as to any of these points, or those on the checklist inside the back cover, she or he must consult a doctor rather than proceed with immunization or deny a child an indicated immunization.

Medical prescription

It is often considered that a written medical prescription is required for a child to commence a course of immunization, especially if immunization is then undertaken by nurses. Such a prescription can conveniently be given at a baby's six-week check.

Nurse immunizing

Nurses may immunize with or without the presence of a doctor as long as they are willing to undertake this professional responsibility and they have had adequate training in all aspects of immunization, including the indications and contra-indications of vaccines, the DOH guidelines, and the recognition and treatment of anaphylaxis. For NHS-employed nurses there should be District Authority policies which the nurse should be aware of and adhere to. Health Visitors should refer to the guidelines on vaccination and immunization issued by the Health Visitors' Association, 50 Southwark Street, London SE1 1UN.

Parental consent

This must be obtained for each and every immunization. Initial written consent, such as that often obtained by the health visitor at the birth visit, is a useful permanent record but is only an agreement for a child to enter a programme of immunization. Presentation of a child for immunization by the family may be seen as consent, though on each occasion parents should be given the relevant details of the immunization to be given and have any questions answered. Particular problems over consent may arise where the immunizers go to the child (e.g. in day nurseries or schools) and special care has to be taken that consent is given in these circumstances.

Parental counselling

Parents often hear incorrect ideas about the infectious diseases and immunization. The nurse or doctor needs to have the right answers to their questions. Some common queries are:

Q. 'There isn't much of these illnesses about these days.'
A. Whooping cough is common, especially during epidemics, and substantial outbreaks occur every four years because immunization fell to below 40 per cent in children born in the 1970s. The same is true for measles because, nationally, uptake is well short of the 90 per cent needed for disease elimination. Rubella-damaged babies still occur, and it is only because British children are immunized against diphtheria, tetanus, and polio that these diseases hardly occur in this country.

Q. 'Only poor children get these illnesses.'
A. The organisms are democratic and can affect any child.

Q. 'I'm going to keep my baby away from other children so he can't catch the germs.'
A. You can never fully protect your child by isolation. Adults and older children can carry some of these illnesses without having any obvious signs of disease.

Q. 'They can treat all these illnesses these days.'

A. Babies still die from whooping cough and 10–20 older children succumb annually to measles, despite having the best hospital treatment. Children who recover can be seriously ill and can suffer from complications which have permanent effects.

Q. 'My child is a year old. Even if he gets one of these illnesses it won't affect him much.'

A. All the illnesses may be serious no matter what the child's age. British children who die from measles usually catch it beyond their early years and it is older unimmunized children who tend to spread whooping cough to babies too young to be protected by immunization.

Q. Immunization is a cause of cot death.

A. This has been looked at by doctors, and found to be untrue.

Q. 'I'm giving my child the homeopathic medicine against whooping cough.'

A. The tests which have been done with this medicine suggest that it does not work. Indeed, it would be very surprising if it did as it is made from the sputum of someone with whooping cough which is then diluted many, many times.

NB: There are other 'folk' remedies for whooping cough which appear to be equally ineffective.

Q. 'These immunizations don't always work.'

A. All the standard childhood immunizations give over 90 per cent protection to children receiving the full course. If a child catches the illness, he or she is likely to have only a mild form.

Q. 'Giving half the dose of immunization is safer, so let's try that first.'

A. Anything less than a full dose may not give protection. A full dose is as safe as a half dose.

Q. 'Babies often get brain damage from the whooping cough injection.'

A. The National Childhood Encephalopathy Study (the most extensive survey of reactions to whooping cough immunization) suggests that the risk of permanent damage from the whooping cough immunization is about once in every 310 000 injections. The risk to an unimmunized child from the disease is currently about six times higher.

Re-evaluation of data from this study suggests that the number of cases of encephalopathy was too small for us to be certain of such an association.

Giving vaccines

Equipment required

Appropriate syringe and needles, spoons;
vaccine to be administered;
toys;
'sharps' container (burn bin);
cotton-wool balls;
shock box (adrenaline, syringe, needles, and airway).

Reconstitution of vaccines and drawing-up

A new needle and syringe must be used for each injection. Many live vaccines are freeze-dried and have to be reconstituted with a diluent provided with the vaccine. It is essential that the appropriate diluent is used. This should be added slowly to the vaccine. Injection with excessive pressure will cause frothing which is thought to make the vaccine less effective. The vaccine solution is then checked to see that it is the correct colour (described in the product insert). If it is not, it should be discarded and the vaccine supplier (e.g. the community pharmacist) notified immediately. Vials of preconstituted vaccines (e.g. DPT) should be shaken to check there is no sediment (the 'shake' test). If there is, the batch of ampoules should be returned to the pharmacy as it may have been frozen at some point and rendered ineffective.

Skin preparation before injection

It is not necessary to swab the skin before injection. However, some immunizers prefer to do so; they should use isopropyl alcohol (Mediswabs, Sterets). For live vaccines (see p. 143 for list) the skin should be allowed to dry (30 seconds is sufficient) before injection, to avoid any possibility of the material used for swabbing the skin killing the vaccine. **Acetone should not be used for pre-injection swabbing: it is highly inflammable and thus a fire hazard.**

Immunization checklist

Preparation

(These activities should preferably be performed out of sight of the parent and child.)

1. The immunizer washes his or her hands.
2. In the clinic a paper towel can be placed on the working surface. When in the patient's home a working surface can be prepared with a clean towel (paper or otherwise).
3. The vaccine expiry date and dosage must be checked.
4. The medical prescription and signature of the parent or guardian are checked (depending on local policy).
5. A 'shock box' for anaphylaxis must be available and its expiry date checked.
6. The syringe and needle are assembled firmly (otherwise the needle can blow off when injecting).
7. If the vaccine is in an ampoule this is broken using a cover (cloth) to protect the fingers. If it is in a rubber-topped vial, the top should be wiped first with a spirit swab. This is followed by waiting for 30 seconds to allow the spirit to evaporate before drawing up the vaccine.
8. Air is expelled carefully from the syringe.

Parents and child

1. The nurse or doctor must first check that the child and the records match and if the accompanying adult is not the parent that they know the child sufficiently well to give a reliable history. The nurse or doctor must then explain the procedure to the child and parent/guardian, check that the injection to be given is indicated, and ask for any appropriate contraindications/special considerations, **especially prior reactions.**
2. The appropriate injection site is then selected in the anterior aspect of the thigh or deltoid muscle of the arm (see Fig. 7) and the child made comfortable (usually, for the younger child on an adult's lap, with one arm, the non-injection arm,

around the adult's waist), removing clothing as necessary, and held firmly so that if he or she flinches the movement will be minimal. Some parents choose not to be present at this point, and it is acceptable for another adult to hold and comfort the child during the actual injection.

Technique

Deep subcutaneous and intramuscular injections

The needle angle for intramuscular injection is 90 degrees to the skin, for subcutaneous injections 45 degrees. Once the needle has been introduced, the piston of the syringe is slightly withdrawn to make certain the needle is not in a blood vessel, then the vaccine is injected gently but steadily. When all has gone the needle is withdrawn. Many immunizers place dry cotton wool on the site

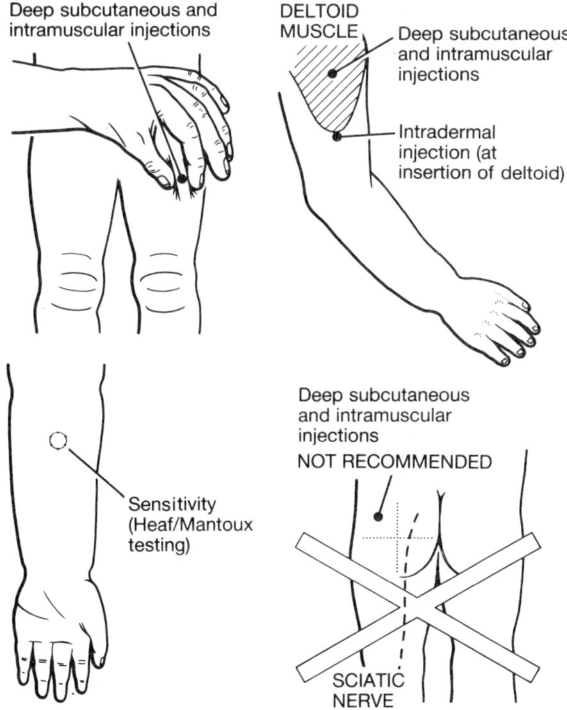

Fig. 7 Sites for vaccination.

and apply gentle pressure or rub for a few moments. A small leakage of vaccine, tissue fluid or blood from the vaccination site is common with sc or im injections and is not a cause for alarm. Cotton wool should be held on the site until the flow stops.

Intradermal injections

(BCG and Mantoux test.) (See Fig. 8.) A short (25 gauge—orange) needle is used. The skin is stretched and the needle inserted slowly with the bevel upwards for 2 mm into the skin almost parallel with the surface. The vaccine is injected cautiously. Resistance should be felt and a white blob begin to rise. **If both do not happen vaccination must stop and the needle be reinserted as it is probably too deep and there is a danger of giving a sub-cutaneous injection.**

After the injection the child is comforted (if necessary) and the parents told about mild reactions and how to manage them. The date when the next injection is due must be worked out with them

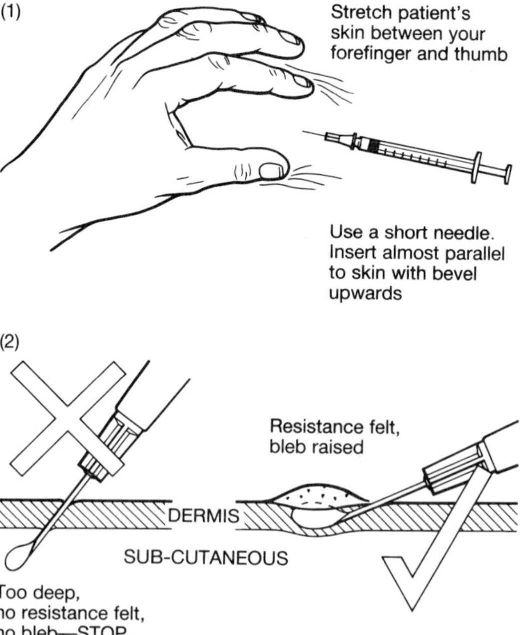

Fig. 8 Intradermal injection technique.

Table 14 Immunization doses (main vaccines only)

Vaccine	Route of administration	Dose	Needle size
Oral polio	Oral	3 drops	Nil
Diphtheria/ tetanus/ Pertussis			
MMR			
Measles	Deep		
Rubella	subcutaneous or	0.5 ml	23G (blue)
Tetanus, diphtheria, or	intramuscular		
pertussis (monovalent)			
low dose diphtheria			
Hepatitis B		0.5 ml	
BCG	Intradermal	0.1 ml (0.05 ml if under 3 months old)	25G (short orange)

For other immunizations, consult manufacturer's product inserts.

and if they have a parent-held immunization record this is best filled in at this point.

Cleansing, replacement, and/or disposal

The needle must not be recapped as this is a potent source of needle-stick injuries. The needle, syringe, and ampoule (after recording the batch number) must all be placed in the burn bin as soon as possible. Empty vaccine packets, syringe packets, and needle caps can be put in an ordinary refuse bin.

Dosage

See Table 14.

Recording immunization

It is vital that immunizations be recorded in central and local records. The precise recording system may vary but the following will be essential as a record of the immunization and that the correct procedure was followed:

Child identification (name, address, date of birth);
Date;
Type of immunization (DPT, Measles, etc.);
Place where immunization given (e.g. Radford Health Centre);
Batch number of vaccine (this may be kept in local records only);
Who gave the injection: a legible signature or printed name.

For the nurse and doctor's protection some District Authorities also suggest in their procedures that the immunizer make records along the lines of 'child fit for immunization—no contraindications'.

Immunization reactions

They are divided into three broad types: mild, severe, and anaphylactic. In addition, there are a few specific to particular immunizations and these are detailed in the descriptions of individual vaccines.

Mild reactions

Parents and older children must be warned to anticipate the commoner mild reactions: mild temperature, headache, general malaise, and local tenderness.

Severe reactions

These can occur after any immunization (or other drug). They are always rare but have been described more often after certain immunizations, most commonly pertussis and influenza. They can be local or general and are defined as:

Local: An extensive area of redness and swelling which becomes indurated (hard) and involves most of the front and side of the thigh, or a major part of the circumference of the upper arm.

General: A fever greater than 39.5°C occurring within 48 hours of injection or any one of the following occurring within 72 hours: anaphylaxis, bronchospasm, laryngeal oedema, generalized collapse, prolonged unresponsiveness, convulsions, or prolonged inconsolable screaming.

Anaphylactic reactions

These are even rarer than severe reactions but can occur after an injection of any drug or immunization, indeed they are much commoner with injected drugs. Though nursing and medical staff are unlikely to see a case of vaccine-induced anaphylaxis in their working life they must be prepared for the situation: first, by checking that adrenalin and the equipment needed to give it are available whenever immunization is taking place; secondly, by knowing how to identify anaphylaxis and to distinguish it from a faint; thirdly, by knowing what action to take should it occur.

The signs of an anaphylactic reaction are of sudden collapse with weak central pulses (femoral or carotid), profuse sweating, and loss of consciousness. Occasionally the onset is more gradual, perhaps with sudden swelling of the skin, wheezing, and difficulty in breathing before collapse. In the case of collapse, it is essential to check first that the child has not simply fainted (common in older vaccinees). This is done by checking the central pulses (carotid in the neck, femoral in the groin). The child or adult who has fainted will be pale but have a strong central pulse. Those worried about their ability to distinguish a faint from anaphylaxis should be reassured by the reports of the few who have seen the latter that they immediately knew what it was. If anaphylaxis is occurring (rapid or gradual onset), a doctor must be summoned **and** adrenalin injected subcutaneously or intramuscularly immediately. If oxygen is available, it should also be given. Nurses and doctors are strongly advised to familiarize themselves with the adrenalin dosages required for emergency therapy (see p. 292).

Reporting reactions

Severe and anaphylactic and other major reactions following immunization must be reported to the local Vaccination and Immunization administration giving:

Name of child and date of birth;
Address of the child;
GP of the child;
Nature of the vaccination;
Vaccine batch number;
The nurse/doctor who immunized;
Date of vaccination;
Where vaccination took place;
Details of the reaction.

A 'Yellow Card' needs to be filled in by a doctor for each severe reaction. This is then sent to the Committee on Safety of Medicines. Severe vaccination reactions brought to accident and emergency departments must also be reported, and the Yellow Card filled in by the doctor examining the child.

The reactions to the standard childhood immunizations are now described.

Triple vaccine: diphtheria/tetanus/pertussis and monovalent pertussis

Mild reactions

Up to 30 per cent of babies have a mild general reaction to immunization, or some 'local' swelling in the 48 hours after injection. Parents may find their baby has a slight temperature, general malaise and/or a red, sore, and swollen injection site. A mild analgesic such as paracetamol may be given. Sometimes a small lump is left after a local reaction; parents can be reassured that this will eventually disappear. These mild reactions are **not** a reason for withholding future pertussis injections.

Severe reactions

These occur only rarely. They can be local or general and are defined as:

Local: An extensive area of redness and swelling which becomes indurated (hard) and involves most of the front and side of the thigh, or a major part of the circumference of the upper arm.

General: A fever greater than 39.5°C occurring within 48 hours of injection or any one of the following occurring within 72 hours:

anaphylaxis, bronchospasm, laryngeal oedema, generalized collapse, prolonged unresponsiveness, convulsions, or prolonged inconsolable screaming.

Neurological damage has been described following pertussis vaccine. This topic is discussed on p. 178.

A baby or child with a severe reaction must be seen by a doctor; the illness may be due to another cause unrelated to the immunization.

If a severe reaction occurs after a Triple or monovalent pertussis immunization, no more injections containing pertussis must be given. If it is not clear if a reaction is mild or severe, a doctor needs to make the final judgement. Details of the reaction need to be entered into the immunization notes. All other indicated injections can be given.

Diphtheria/tetanus, monovalent diphtheria, and tetanus

Mild local reactions occur in young children following these vaccines but are less common than with pertussis. Reactions are more frequent and painful in older children, particularly with diphtheria vaccine (the reason for this is not clear) and after the tenth birthday a low-dose vaccine is given (see p. 164). Severe local and general reactions have been described, but are much rarer than with pertussis-containing vaccines in pre-school children.

MMR and measles

A mild general reaction 6–11 days after the injection occurs in a quarter to a third of children. There is occasionally a temperature and rash lasting up to 48 hours. The child is not infectious to other children. Very occasionally the fever may trigger a febrile convulsion. Children have also shown mild facial swelling 3–4 weeks after immunization. Severe reactions are extremely rare.

Polio

Extremely rarely the vaccine may revert to its wild type and invade the nervous system (see p. 183).

Rubella

A few girls very occasionally experience some temporary joint pains as well as, or instead of, a mild general reaction (headache and feeling unwell). Severe reactions are extremely rare.

BCG

Mild reactions

There is normally a response at the vaccination site commencing within 2–6 weeks. Usually this is a small lump that enlarges and discharges some fluid to leave an ulcer. If this happens, a dry dressing should be applied but allowing air to the skin as this hastens healing. The discharge is not a source of tuberculosis to others. Children can go swimming though some authorities recommend an air-tight dressing while in the water. Some swelling and aching of the glands in the armpit often occurs temporarily. Deep ulcers are usually due to the BCG being given too deeply.

Severe reactions

Severe local reactions, suppurative adenitis, and osteomyelitis rarely occur following BCG and may be long delayed after the immunization. These must be brought to the attention of the doctor who may decide to consult an appropriate specialist with regard to therapy.

Individual immunizations

Not every vaccine available in the UK is covered in this section. For example, those used exclusively for adults, such as anthrax, will not be found here.

Those used only for travelling abroad are covered in the section on travel abroad.

Cholera immunization

Inactivated vaccine

Preparation

This is a heat-inactivated suspension of sub-types of *Vibrio cholerae* type 01.

Effectiveness

The vaccine is relatively ineffective in protecting individuals, and plays even less role in controlling infection at the community level. What limited protection is afforded lasts only 3–6 months.

Indications

The vaccine is scarcely ever indicated for any children. One or two countries still require certificated evidence of immunization (Niger and Qatar in 1988), though a single dose will suffice for this. Individuals are often given incorrect advice that they should have such protection.

Contraindications

Acute febrile illness or substantial chronic illness; age under one year; pregnancy; previous severe local or general reactions to a prior cholera injection.

How given and dosage

Im or deep sc injection. Children from 12 months to 4 yr are given a first dose of 0.1 ml, with subsequent doses of 0.3 ml; those aged five to nine, a first dose of 0.3 ml and subsequent doses of 0.5 ml; those aged over 10, a first dose of 0.5 ml and subsequent doses of 1.0 ml.

Reactions

Mild local reactions are common; general reactions very rare.

Diphtheria immunization

Inactivated vaccine

Immunization strategy

Protection of all susceptibles. The target is for 90 per cent of all children to have had three doses (within the Triple vaccine) by the age of six months.

Preparation

Diphtheria toxoid, preferably in its adsorbed form. This is normally given combined with tetanus and pertussis vaccines (Triple) but is also available with tetanus alone or on its own. A special low-dose monovalent preparation is available for adults and children beyond their tenth birthday.

Effectiveness

This is very high. The disease is confined to unimmunized individuals, although mild illness or asymptomatic infection may still occur.

Indications

All children

Every child should commence diphtheria immunization at two months and continue as per the national schedule (see back cover).

Unimmunized individuals

Older children (and adults) who have not been previously protected should receive the low dose diphtheria vaccine, three times at monthly intervals.

Contraindications

Acute febrile illness is a reason for deferring immunization for one week. Immunization should not proceed when there has been a severe reaction to a preceding dose.

How given

Im or deep sc injection.

Dosage

0.5 ml alone or as a combined preparation.

Reactions

These are extremely uncommon—usually local reddening with mild constitutional upset.

Notes

Booster doses for adults may be necessary as immunity from childhood immunization may not persist into adult life. If the person is going to a country where diphtheria is endemic, or there is a risk from exposure in an outbreak, it may be desirable to boost immunity by use of the low-dose vaccine.

Hepatitis A immunization

Immunization strategy

Prevention of outbreaks in institutions, and among travellers to all countries except Northern Europe, North America, and Australia and New Zealand.

Preparations

Passive immunization

For close contacts of patients living in institutions, human normal immunoglobulin (HNIG) is protective in the following doses—under 10 years 250 mg, over 10 years 500 mg.

For children under the age of 10 travelling abroad for 2 months, 125 mg should be given, for 3–5 months 250 mg. The dose is doubled in older children and adults.

Because HNIG may interfere with the development of immunity from live virus vaccines, a gap of 3 weeks should be left between active immunization and administration of HNIG. If HNIG has been given live vaccines should not be given for 3 months.

Hepatitis B immunization

Inactivated vaccine

Immunization strategy

Prevention of perinatal transmission and protection of high risk susceptibles.

Preparations

Passive immunization

for immediate protection is afforded by hepatitis B immunoglobulin (HBIG) given as soon as possible after exposure and repeated one month later—now usually combined with hepatitis B vaccine (HBVac).

Active immunization

Two types of vaccine are available, each containing 20 microgram/ml of HBsAg adsorbed on aluminium hydroxide adjuvant: (a) purified from human plasma, in such a way as to inactivate Hepatitis B virus and HIV, H-B-Vax, Merck Sharp and Dohme; (b) produced by genetic engineering using a recombinant DNA technique, (Engerix B, Smith, Kline, and French).

Effectiveness

Combined passive and active immunizations are highly effective in preventing vertical transmission from mother to child. Active immunization is 90 per cent effective in providing protection to children, somewhat less for adults.

Indications and types of immunization given

Preventing perinatal transmission

—both active and passive immunization. Infants born to mothers known to be carriers of HBsAg (a component of the hepatitis B virus) should receive HB vac. Mothers who are known to be HBeAg positive (core antigen positive) and anti-HBe negative (core antibody negative) are highly infectious and their infants should receive HBIG in addition to the vaccine. The following groups have a higher rate of hepatitis B infection and should be screened during pregnancy: ethnic groups other than Caucasian women who have lived outside Europe, North America, Australia, and New Zealand; all those where the history suggests increased risk of hepatitis B virus infection (principally intravenous drug abusers), and mothers with a recent history of hepatitis B infection.

Protecting individuals exposed to infected blood (eg needle-stick injury)

—both active and passive immunization.

Protecting susceptibles

—active immunization.
Susceptible groups include the following:

Children and adults entering residential institutions for the mentally handicapped where there are known to be carriers of a higher prevalence of hepatitis B virus.

Children and adults with chronic renal disease who are awaiting dialysis or transplantation. In immunosuppressed patients the immune response is likely to be poor so these patients should be protected as soon as they are considered for dialysis or transplant.

Health-care staff: doctors, dentists, nurses, midwives, and others involved for more than six months in direct patient care of individuals suspected to be at higher risk of infection, especially staff who have direct contact with blood and body fluids through the use of, or contact with, needles and other sharp instruments. Immunization is particularly recommended for those working in units caring for known carriers of hepatitis B; laboratory workers and mortuary technicians; the staff of residential institutions for the mentally handicapped (unless the risk is known to be low by serological testing); health workers (including students) involved in patient care in parts of the world with increased prevalence of hepatitis B (for practical purposes all less developed countries).

Haemophiliacs and those receiving regular blood transfusions or blood products.

Some adult groups: active homosexuals and injecting drug abusers, if known to be non-immune.

Contraindications

1. Acute febrile illness is a reason for delaying active but not passive immunization.
2. There is no point in giving Hepatitis B vaccine to individuals who are already carriers (HBsAg positive).

How given and dosage

Active and passive immunization

—used following exposure to HBsAg-positive blood, eg where there is a risk of perinatal transmission or through needle-stick injury.

For newborn infants and children under 10 years, give H-B-Vac (MSD) 0.5 ml (10 microgram) im (anterolateral thigh or deltoid), repeated at one month and six months after exposure (intradermal use **not** recommended) or Engerix B (Smith, Kline, and French) 0.5 ml using the same procedure at similar time intervals; plus HBIG 2.0 ml (200 mg) im (contralateral thigh or deltoid) as soon as possible after exposure. For perinatal infection HBIG should be given less than 12 hours after birth. Because of uncertainty about persistence of immunity in these children, it has been recommended that a booster dose is repeated at 5-yearly intervals.

For children over 10 years (and adults) give HBVac 1.0 ml (20 microgram) im (deltoid is preferred site) repeated at one month and six months after exposure (alternatively, 0.1 ml (2 microgram) intradermally*) plus HBIG 5.0 ml (500 mg) im (contralateral arm or thigh; buttock may be used with special care in view of large volume) as soon as possible after exposure.

Active immunization

Give vaccine 1.0 ml (20 microgram) im repeated after one month and six months to children over 10, and 0.5 ml (10 microgram) im repeated after one month and six months to children under 10. For rapid immunization, the third dose can be given two months after the initial dose with a booster at 12 months. In patients with haemophilia the intradermal or subcutaneous route may be used.

Reactions

Apart from a mild constitutional upset and some soreness and redness at the site of injection, no serious side-effects have been reported.

Notes

1. Intradermal injection

While the intradermal route for immunization is economically attractive for group vaccination as less vaccine will be used, the immune response may not be satisfactory should this more difficult injection technique not be carried out correctly. If this route is used, it would seem sensible to check the antibody response by serological testing.

2. Immunodeficient children

The Hepatitis B vaccine is safe for use in patients who are immunodeficient or immunosuppressed but the antibody response may be poor. An increased dose of the vaccine may be necessary to improve protection, and the serological response should be checked.

3. HIV risk

No HIV (or hepatitis) infection has been attributed to the vaccine prepared from human plasma and there is no risk of infection from the genetically engineered vaccine.

* Not yet recommended by the manufacturer but practised by some doctors.

4. Post-immunization check

Some individuals do not respond to vaccination and, if risk of exposure is high, immunity should be checked 3 months after completing the immunization course.

Influenza immunization

Inactivated vaccine

Immunization strategy

Protection of children with chronic respiratory and cardiac disease. Each year recommendations are made as to what strains should be included in the vaccines designed to provide some protection for the coming winter. The precise vaccine may, therefore, vary from year to year. Immunization is best carried out during the late summer or early autumn. The vaccines will not control epidemics and are recommended only for those at high risk.

Preparation

Vaccines are grown on chicken embryos and then inactivated. The precise composition varies from year to year.

Effectiveness

Current influenza vaccines produce reasonably good immunity, and are safe, being associated with only mild side effects.

Indications

Chronic lung and heart disease

Children with underlying chronic conditions involving the lungs (cystic fibrosis, severe asthma, and bronchopulmonary dysplasia) and heart (many forms of congenital heart disease). Immunization should be considered in children undergoing treatment for malignant conditions, including leukaemia during epidemics.

This is not done under the age of six months and is most commonly offered when the child enters school or day nursery where he will be in contact with a large number of other children.

Contraindications

1. Acute febrile illness is a reason for deferring immunization for one week.
2. Severe egg allergy. As the virus strains for vaccine production are grown in developing chick embryos severe egg allergy—angio-oedema, urticaria, acute respiratory distress, and collapse—is a contraindication.
3. Age under six months. No data are available on the use of influenza vaccine in infants under six months of age and they are not normally immunized.

How given

Primary immunization (6 months and older): two injections (0.5 ml) with an interval of 4–6 weeks. A booster injection should be given each year. When the recommended vaccine changes, only one injection is needed if prior immunizations have been received.

Reactions

Mild systemic and local reactions to the vaccine occur in up to 10 per cent of recipients, usually within the 6–48 hours after immunization. More severe reactions are uncommon.

Notes

1. Immunosuppressed children

Children who are no longer receiving chemotherapy are likely to have an adequate response with a high rate of seroconversion. If children are still receiving chemotherapy, the immune response is likely to be poor. The optimum time to protect children with malignant disease who must still continue their treatments is when they have been off chemotherapy for 3–4 weeks and when they have neutrophil and lymphocyte counts over $1000/mm^3$.

2. Kawasaki disease or chronic arthritis

If these children require long-term aspirin therapy, influenza immunization should be considered because it is thought these children, if they acquire influenza, are at increased risk of developing Reye's syndrome.

Measles/mumps/rubella immunization (MMR)

Live vaccine

Immunization strategy

Protection of all susceptibles and national elimination of the measles, mumps, and rubella viruses. The target is for 90 per cent of children to be immunized by their second birthday, with similar or better levels among school entrants.

Following MMR's successful use in the United States and parts of Europe as a method of protecting susceptibles and minimizing the circulation of the three viruses, the vaccine was introduced nationally in October 1988. It had been successfully tried out in three Health Districts (two in England, one in Scotland). The successful introduction of MMR was crucial for the control of measles and rubella. Individual districts and general practitioners had achieved the target of 90 per cent, but nationally measles immunization has only just reached 70 per cent. By April 1989, 80 per cent of children had received MMR by their second birthday. The policy of selective female immunization against rubella although producing a higher uptake had reached the limits of its effectiveness, and an intolerable number of terminations for exposure to rubella still having to be performed (see p. 104). Any further reduction in the number of rubella-damaged fetuses requires the reinforcement afforded by vaccination of children of both sexes in their second year of life, which with high uptake will reduce virus circulation. Also, mumps is a continuing source of substantial child and adult morbidity (see p. 91).

Since the peak ages for catching all three diseases involve the pre-school and early school years, it is essential to immunize as many children as possible in these age groups, otherwise virus elimination may take many years. This kind of coverage will be achieved by initially immunizing with MMR both at 15 months and at the same time as the pre-school booster (age 4–5 years). Children (and adults) who have already had measles, mumps, or rubella, and children who have already been immunized with measles (or rubella) vaccine, can all be immunized with MMR. There is no harm from 'double immunization'. As elimination of the virus will take time the policy of immunizing secondary schoolgirls and all sero-negative women must also continue in the immediate future.

Preparation

The freeze-dried vaccine contains three attenuated live viruses. Three vaccines are available: Pluserix-MMR (Smith, Kline, and French), Schwartz strain measles, RA27/3 rubella, and Urabe Am/9 mumps; MMR 11 (Wellcome), further attenuated Enders Edmonston strain: measles RA27/3 rubella, and Jery/Lynn mumps; and Immravax (Merieux), Schwarz strain measles, RA27/3 rubella, and Urabe Am/9 mumps. The measles, mumps, and rubella components are currently available in Britain in their monovalent forms.

Effectiveness

All individual components give long-lasting individual protection following a single immunization. (For measles and rubella this has been shown to last at least 20 years.) Effectiveness seems equally high when the vaccines are given together.

Indications

Children aged 1–2 years

MMR is given to children of both sexes in the second year of life.

Children aged 4–5 years (pre-school booster)

MMR is offered to children of both sexes at the time of their pre-school booster if they have not received this previously. This will entail two separate injections, MMR and diphtheria/tetanus (and polio drops). When parents are reluctant for two injections to be given together MMR should take preference and the diphtheria/tetanus should be given later.

Children between two and four years, older children and adults
These can be given MMR.

Contraindications

1. Acute febrile illness is a reason for deferring immunization for one week.
2. Children with immunodeficient conditions must not receive MMR. This does not apply to HIV children, see p. 217). Siblings of immunocompromised children can be given MMR.
3. A history of extreme sensitivity to neomycin or kanamycin is a contraindication because the vaccine contains traces of these antibiotics (see p. 145).
4. A history of anaphylaxis following exposure to chicken or egg products is a contraindication (but not the commoner forms of egg allergy: rash, diarrhoea). This is because the measles component is prepared on chicken fibroblasts and the mumps on chicken fibroblasts or egg amniotic fluid.
5. Pregnancy. Though no cases of fetal abnormalities have been reported as due to any of the vaccine strains, it is recommended not to immunize in pregnancy. If it happens inadvertently, it is not an indication for termination of the pregnancy.

How given

A single sc or im injection.

Dosage

0.5 ml.

Reactions

Reactions are very similar to those following the present measles vaccination with a mild fever, malaise, and/or rash occurring in a quarter to a third of children, commonly in the period 6–11 days after injection, and lasting about 48 hours. The rash, if it occurs, follows a day or so after the fever and looks like that of rubella. The family should be warned to anticipate these reactions and told about temperature management (see Note 1 below). It should also be explained to them that the child with such a reaction is non-infectious. Children have also occasionally shown mild facial swelling 2–3 weeks after immunization, presumably due to the mumps component.

There have been occasional reports of mumps encephalitis occurring within 28 days of immunization, and in a few of these the vaccine virus has been identified in the CSF. All have recovered without long-term sequelae. Data are still being collected to establish the true incidence of this reaction, but it is likely to be something of the order of 1 in 1 million immunizations.

Notes

1. Child with a personal or close (first-degree relatives) family history of convulsions

These children must be immunized as they are at high risk of a convulsion when they catch measles, particularly if their history is of febrile convulsions. There is a much smaller risk (one-eighth to one-tenth) that a febrile reaction due to the immunization could also trigger a convulsion. Parents of such a child must be advised on temperature management when immunization takes place. If a temperature develops, various strategies can be employed depending on the severity of the convulsive tendency. Where risk is small, a combination of oral paracetamol, removing excess clothes, and keeping the room cool is usually effective.

The previous practice of administering immunoglobulin simultaneously with the injection must now be discontinued as this may limit the effectiveness of the mumps and rubella components of the vaccine.

2. Parent education

Since the MMR vaccine is new to families, there will be particular advantages in giving parents leaflets explaining its rationale and its associated mild reactions.

3. Exposure to measles—a measles outbreak

If a child is thought to have been exposed to measles and has not previously been immunized, then an injection of MMR given within 72 hours of exposure will lessen the impact of the disease.

Measles immunization

Live vaccine

Preparation

A monovalent live attenuated virus.

This vaccine should now only be used where parents refuse MMR but still wish their child to have protection against measles. Contraindications are as specified for MMR (p. 174).

Mumps immunization

Live vaccine

Preparation

A monovalent live attenuated virus.

This vaccine has few indications for its use in isolation. Where parents specifically wish their child to be protected against mumps they should be strongly advised to use MMR vaccine.

Pertussis immunization

Inactivated vaccine

Immunization strategy

Protection of individuals and limitation of epidemics by high herd immunity. Target is for 90 per cent of all children to have had three doses (within the Triple vaccine) by age of six months.

Preparation

A suspension of killed *B. pertussis* organisms, either combined with dipththeria and tetanus (Triple vaccine) or as a monovalent vaccine.

Effectiveness

Highly effective in protecting individuals from disease. One dose gives approximately 30 per cent protection; two, 60 per cent; three, 90 per cent. Disease is milder in those few who are infected after immunization.

Indications

All children

Every child should commence pertussis immunization at two months and continue as per the national schedule (see back cover).

Unimmunized individuals

Older children who have not been previously protected against pertussis should receive pertussis vaccine (either monovalent or combined, as appropriate) especially when younger children are at risk.

Contraindications

1. Acute febrile illness is a reason for deferring immunization for one week.
2. A severe local or general reaction to a prior immunization including pertussis. Definitions:

Local: An extensive area of redness and swelling which becomes indurated and involves most of the front and side surface of the thigh or a major part of the circumference of the upper arm.
General: Any of: temperature over 39.5°C within 48 hours, anaphylaxis, bronchospasm, laryngeal oedema, generalized collapse, prolonged unresponsiveness, convulsions, or prolonged inconsolable screaming occurring within 72 hours of immunization.

How given

By im or deep sc injection.

Dosage

0.5 ml, alone or as a combined vaccine.

Reactions

Mild reactions (irritability, local tenderness, and pyrexia) are common: 5–30 per cent depending on criteria. These are commoner with the second and third dose; however, it does not necessarily follow that a child who has had a mild reaction to one dose will react to following injections. A small, firm nodule frequently develops at the injection site. Parents can be reassured that this will either resolve or become impalpable as the arm grows. Severe reactions are uncommon but are considered more likely to re-occur. A connection between pertussis immunization and handicapping reactions (brain damage) was suggested by the national childhood encephalopathy study, though with a very low frequency (one case per 310 000 injections, a rate equivalent to once every 1500 GP or health-visitor working years) **re-evaluation of this data has suggested that this data is inconclusive and there is no causative association.** It seems that in the well-reported cases where pertussis vaccine was thought to have caused damage, vaccination has happened to coincide with the sudden onset of brain disease. Parents concerned about the vaccine need this to be explained and to be reminded that complications after whooping cough are, in contrast, relatively common.

Notes

1. Children with problem histories

(1) Children with a documented history of cerebral damage in the neonatal period;

(2) children with a personal history of convulsions;

(3) children whose parents or siblings have a history of idiopathic epilepsy.

Though the chances of reactions may be higher in immunizing these children, they should still be protected as benefits outweigh the risks. Parents of children in categories (2) and (3) should be instructed in methods of fever control (paracetamol, stripping) so as to reduce the risk of a febrile convulsion. The Joint Committee on Vaccination and Immunization and the BPA Committee for Immunization and Infectious Diseases are agreed that paracetamol is as likely to be as efficacious and safe in a 2-months-old as in a 3-months-old child.

Where the nurse or doctor is unsure as to whether to give pertussis or not they should rapidly seek specialist advice (preferably by phone) rather than deny the child protection.

2. Mythical contraindications

These are legion for pertussis (see p. 146).

3. Cerebral irritation and a history of convulsions

are no longer considered contraindications.

4. Stable neurological conditions

Children with stable handicaps (e.g. cerebral palsy or spina bifida) may be immunized.

5. Prior illness

Certain virus infections may result in an illness similar to pertussis (parapertussis). A child reported to have had pertussis need not be immunized if the diagnosis was confirmed by detection or isolation of *B. pertussis* (see p. 130).

6. Neurodegenerative conditions

It would seem wise not to immunize children with such conditions against pertussis. Note: children covered by Notes 4 and 6 will all be known to paediatricians and there will be value in discussing individual cases.

7. Oral homeopathic vaccine

This is prepared from the sputum of a pertussis sufferer. Having had multiple dilutions it probably does no harm but the evidence from the single published trial is that there is no protective effect.

Pneumococcal immunization

Inactivated vaccine

Immunization strategy

Given to individuals with conditions making them susceptible to severe pneumococcal infections. In normal adults and children the spleen makes a substantial contribution to protection against pneumococci. Children with absent or ineffective spleens are therefore susceptible.

Preparation

A capsular polysaccharide (cell-wall) extract of 23 sub-types of *Streptococcus pneumoniae*, known as Pneumovax II.

Effectiveness

The vaccine is relatively successful in preventing severe pneumococcal infections (pneumonia, meningitis, bacteraemia) in susceptible children beyond their second birthday. Antibody levels remain high for at least five years. It is ineffective under two years and no protection is afforded against commoner conditions where pneumococcus is sometimes implicated (recurrent otitis media).

It is recommended that prophylactic antibiotics are used in addition to immunization in children at risk of pneumococcal infections.

Indications

Children with absent or deficient spleens

Children beyond their second birthday (and adults) with any condition involving lack of the spleen or loss of splenic function: sickle-cell disease (not trait), nephrotic syndrome, some immunodeficiency states, post splenectomy.

Contraindications

Acute febrile illness is a reason for deferring immunization for one week.

How given

A single dose by im or deep sc injection. Boosters may be required at 5-yearly intervals. When splenectomy is planned, vaccination should take place at least two weeks before this.

Dosage

0.5 ml.

Reactions

About half of vaccinees report mild local symptoms. One per cent have fever, myalgia, or more severe local reactions. Anaphylactic-like reactions are extremely rare (estimated one per 200 000 doses).

Notes

1. Specialist consultation

Any child who might benefit from protection is likely to be known to a paediatrician, who should be consulted prior to immunization.

Polio (OPV) immunization

Live oral vaccine

Immunization strategy

Protection of all individuals and minimizing wild (pathogenic) virus circulation in the community by high herd-immunity. Target is for 90 per cent of all children to have had three doses by the age of six months.

Preparation

Live attenuated vaccine combining the three strains of polio virus.

Effectiveness

Immunization gives protection both in the gut and systemically. The former reduces symptomless excretion and reduces circulation of wild virus. The three doses protect 95 per cent of individuals against the three strains of virus.

Indications

All children

Every child should commence polio immunization at two months as per the national schedule (see back cover).

Unimmunized individuals

All older unimmunized children and adults should use a catch-up schedule.

Previously immunized children and adults

travelling to endemic areas who have not had a booster in the preceding 10 years should be given one before travelling.

Contraindications

1. Acute febrile illness is a reason for deferring immunization for one week.
2. Immunodeficiency in a child, their siblings, or parents are contraindications and IPV is given instead because of the concern that the child or deficient family member would be at risk of infection from a live vaccine.

   HIV-positive children can be immunized with OPV in safety. HIV infection acquired from the mother during pregnancy cannot be confirmed until the child is 15 months old, long after the primary immunization course has been completed. If either parent has symptomatic HIV infection, IPV is recommended.
3. A child suffering from **acute diarrhoea** should have immunization delayed. However, vaccination should proceed if there is merely chronic loose stools (toddler diarrhoea).
4. Extreme antibiotic sensitivity. OPV contains traces of neomycin, streptomycin, and penicillin (though less than is sometimes found in doorstep milk). In the very rare circumstance of extreme hypersensitivity (anaphylactic) to these antibiotics a child should not receive OPV.
5. Pregnancy. There is no evidence of OPV ever having caused fetal damage. It is, however, advised not to be given to a pregnant woman in the first four months of pregnancy (though her children may be immunized). If there is a

compelling reason (e.g. an unprotected woman travelling to an endemic country), IPV should be given.

How given

The vaccine is given orally, with three drops constituting a dose. It is customary in schoolchildren to put the drops on sugar lumps. When this is done care must be taken that large numbers of lumps are not prepared in advance as some may be left in the warm for so long that the vaccine is inactivated.

Dosage

3 drops.

Reactions

Very occasionally (approximately once every 1–5 million doses) OPV will revert to its wild form in the vaccinee and result in poliomyelitis in the child or a close contact.

Notes

1. Breast feeding

This does not interfere with vaccination.

2. Immunizing parents

It is impractical to immunize adults in child health clinics (Where is the immunization record kept?) and unprotected adults should be given the vaccine by their general practitioner.

3. Combining with inactivated polio vaccine (IPV)

Children from other countries and some adults will have had IPV. For purposes of completing courses and boosters IPV and OPV can be seen as interchangeable, and an adult who had IPV as a child and needs a booster can have a single dose of OPV.

Polio (IPV) immunization

Inactivated vaccine

Preparation

An inactivated combination of the three polio virus strains.

Inactivated polio vaccine (IPV) is used in the UK normally, only for immunodeficient individuals. It is also recommended for family contacts of such children. Although OPV can be given to HIV-positive children, IPV is recommended when there are symptomatic HIV family members. Other countries use it more extensively amongst healthy children. It is safe and gives good individual protection, though it may be less successful in preventing wild virus circulation. Like OPV it combines the three virus strains. It is given by im or sc injection as per the OPV schedule, but with only febrile illness, pregnancy, and extreme antibiotic hypersensitivity as contraindications. It is essentially interchangeable with OPV so that someone commencing a course with one vaccine may complete it with the other.

Dosage

0.5 ml.

Rubella immunization

Live vaccine

Immunization strategy

The protection of all susceptibles. The UK has adopted the MMR vaccine and so reinforced current rubella immunization strategy with disease elimination. However, the schoolgirl immunization programme, routine blood-testing of adult women, and postnatal immunization of seronegative women will need to continue. A decision will be made later this decade as to whether schoolgirl immunization will be required. This will depend on the MMR uptake rate, and on continued evidence from the USA where MMR has been given for about 20 years, that immunity to rubella persists into adulthood.

Preparation

This is a live attenuated freeze-dried vaccine grown on human diploid cells.

Effectiveness

A single dose is considered to give protection for at least 20 years. Even though antibody levels decline over this period, there seems to be no fall in protection. A few women do not sero-convert (see Note 4 below).

Indications

All girls between their tenth and fourteenth birthdays

These children are usually immunized at school or in the GP surgery. A prior history of rubella infection is not a contraindication.

Seronegative women of child-bearing age

It is essential that all women in this age-group be tested for rubella antibodies.

Seronegative male and female hospital staff

This is to protect susceptible pregnant women in antenatal clinics. All health-service staff should therefore be screened for their immunological status.

Contraindications

1. Acute febrile illness is a reason for deferring immunization for one week.
2. Immunodeficient children and adults must not be immunized.

3. Pregnancy is a contraindication. Some previous vaccines (now out of use in the UK) were considered teratogenic (producing malformations). However, their use has been discontinued and no malformations have been reported with the diploid vaccines in cases of immunization of susceptible pregnant women. Hence, although pregnancy remains a contraindication (at least a month should elapse between immunization and pregnancy), termination of pregnancy is **not** indicated when immunization inadvertently occurs.
4. Extreme antibiotic sensitivity to neomycin or polymixin is a contraindication (see p. 145).

How given

A single im or deep sc injection.

Dosage

0.5 ml.

Reactions

Mild joint pains are common, occurring in up to 20 per cent of adults receiving vaccines but only 3 per cent of children. They commence any time from 3 to 25 days after injection (most commonly 8–14 days) and usually last 2–4 days. Mild general reactions are also common, with fever, sore throat, lymphadenopathy, and rashes. These are mild infections and are therefore delayed in onset. Mild transient neuropathies ('pins and needles') have also been reported, but more severe reactions are extremely rare.

Notes

1. Prior history of rubella

Diagnosis of rubella is often problematic and such a history is never a justification for withholding immunization for children. In a woman beyond her sixteenth birthday, policy is to check her rubella serology unless it seems likely that she will not return later. In that case immunization should be given without serology.

2. Children with joint conditions

Mild joint pain is a common reaction following rubella immunization, and exacerbation of childhood arthritis has been reported. Hence, it is worthwhile testing the rubella serology of any girl with such a condition prior to immunization (blood tests are usually being done anyway) as she may have achieved natural immunity. However, if the girl is non-immune she should be immunized.

3. Co-ordination of school and GP immunization

Secondary schoolgirls may be immunized in either setting. However, whenever a girl reports to one agency that she has been or will be immunized by the other this must be verified, so that evasion of immunization may be detected.

4. Negative serology despite prior immunization

Routine blood tests may fail to detect low antibody levels which still are protective for the fetus. If there is a history of immunization, the problem needs to be explained to the woman and the case discussed with a specialist.

5. Postnatal immunization

Some seronegative women are detected in pregnancy by antenatal screening. They will need immunization after delivery. This can be done in the postnatal ward or at a postnatal check, unless a transfusion has been given in which case immunization should be delayed for three months. If anti-D (rhesus) immunoglobulin is also needed, the two can be given simultaneously at different sites.

6. Information for women

All women who are tested should be informed of their results in writing.

7. Immigrant women

Few less developed countries offer rubella immunization, and women from these countries have been shown to be more often unprotected than their UK-born counterparts. This group therefore requires special attention.

Tetanus immunization

Inactivated vaccine

Immunization strategy

Protection of all susceptibles. Target is for 90 per cent of all children to have had three doses (within the Triple vaccine) by the age of six months.

Preparation

A cell-free suspension of the inactivated adsorbed toxin of tetanus, produced either on its own, combined with diphtheria and pertussis (DTP or Triple Vaccine), or with diphtheria alone. A plain form of vaccine is available but this is less immunogenic and has no advantage over the adsorbed type.

Indications

All children

Every child should commence tetanus immunization at two months and continue as per the national schedule (see back cover).

Unimmunized individuals

Unimmunized older children and adults should receive protection using a catch-up schedule.

Following injury

See p. 215 in Practical immunization: questions and answers for a detailed discussion.

Contraindications

Acute febrile illness is a reason for delaying routine vaccination but vaccine should be given immediately if the indication is an injury.

How given

By im or deep sc injection.

Effectiveness

This is very high. Disease is now confined to the unimmunized. Immunity of pregnant mothers is transferred to the fetus and prevents neonatal tetanus. The adsorbed form is marginally more effective in conferring immunity than the plain preparation.

Reactions

Mild local reactions are common, especially in older children and adults. These can arise soon after injection or up to 10 days later. They may persist for a few days and require an analgesic, such as paracetamol. If the injection has been superficial, a nodule may be felt. This will eventually resolve. General reactions are uncommon and anaphylactic responses exceedingly rare.

Notes

1. Excessive number of doses

Since hypersensitivity reactions can occur, individuals should not receive large numbers of doses. Unless there is high risk of exposure, an adult need not be immunized at less than 10-yearly intervals.

2. Severe local reaction

This suggests good immunity and probably no further doses are needed for at least 10 years. Some practitioners will first try skin testing with a dilute dose, but this is an unreliable method of determining sensitivity to the vaccine.

Tuberculosis (BCG) immunization

Live vaccine

Immunization strategy

Protection of all susceptibles. Target is for 95 per cent of secondary schoolchildren to be tuberculin positive. With declining disease incidence the broad mass of schoolchildren are at decreasing risk; however, present policy is to continue routine school immunization. Incidence is also declining amongst Asian and African families but remains at a higher level than for the rest of the population. If routine immunization ceases, a programme will still be needed in every Health District for these groups.

Preparation

BCG (Bacillus Calmette–Guerin) in a freeze-dried preparation form. BCG is an attenuated mycobacterium (the family of bacteria causing tuberculosis).

Effectiveness

BCG is moderately effective. In adolescents, 70 per cent protection is given for 15 years. The degree of protection afforded by BCG given in the neonatal period is less certain, though it is thought to prevent TB spreading through the blood-stream and, in particular, to protect against TB meningitis.

Indications

High-risk neonates

This is done without prior sensitivity testing for all newborn infants (see HIV-positive children, p. 217) in contact with infectious cases of respiratory TB, or in families of ethnic Asian or African origin (not West Indian), or countries where TB is more prevalent (for practical purposes all less-developed countries), and when there is history of TB in a family member during the previous 5 years. **In all other circumstances the child must be shown to be tuberculin negative before giving BCG.**

Some children acquire BCG immunity naturally. They do not need BCG and if they receive it can suffer a severe local reaction. This can be tested by seeing if the child's skin is sensitive to tuberculin, an inactive derivative of the TB organism. Groups to be tested and if tuberculin (Heaf/Mantoux) negative given BCG: schoolchildren between the ages of 10 and 13 years; close contacts of cases of infectious acute respiratory TB; health-service staff; students, including those in teacher-training.

Contraindications

1. Acute febrile illness is a reason for deferring immunization for one week.
2. Tuberculin-positive individuals.
3. Immunodeficiency (see p. 218), including symptomatic or asymptomatic HIV infection—this includes new-born and young babies of HIV mothers.
4. Generalized severe septic skin conditions.
5. Pregnancy. No cases of malformation have been reported. Where immunization inadvertently occurs, this is **not** a reason for advising termination of pregancy.

How given—sensitivity testing

Uses PPD (purified protein derivative). This is used for diagnosis and contact tracing. For the latter two, interpretation is difficult and requires specialist consultation.

Mantoux testing

(Suitable for individual patients.) Use 1 : 1000 dilution (100 u/ml). PPD given as an intradermal injection (Fig. 8, p. 156). Inject 0.1 ml.

Use only one needle and syringe per patient.

Heaf multiple puncture test

(Suitable for mass testing.) This uses a spring-loading 'gun' with six short needles set at 1 mm until a child reaches their second birthday, 2 mm thereafter. The PPD dilution (100 000 u/ml) is more concentrated than for the Mantoux test and is specially supplied in vials sufficient for about 50 tests. A variety of applicators may be used: a sterile platinum-wire loop, a sterile glass-rod, or a syringe and needle. With one of these a very small amount of PPD is put on the forearm (see Fig. 7 for site, p. 000). The applicator itself should not touch the skin. If it does, then re-disinfection (loop or rod) or changing (needle) is needed. The PPD is smoothed on the skin using the loaded 'gun' end-plate. The end-plate is held firmly at 90° on the skin and the 'gun' then fired. The needles of the 'gun' must be kept sharp and the 'gun' end-plate disinfected between each person by dipping it with its needles in spirit and then passing these through a flame so that the spirit on the apparatus catches light and heat sterilization takes place. The gun should not be kept in the flame and it must be allowed to cool before the next child! This will take about 30 seconds. The gun must not become contaminated in this time. If necessary, it can be protected in a sterile tube. (Note: some Health Districts now use disposable heads for guns, removing any need for flaming.)

Interpreting the Mantoux

Read between 72 and 96 hours. A positive result is an **indurated** (hard) area of 6 mm or more diameter.

Interpreting the Heaf

Read between 72 hours and 10 days. Positive reactions are those of Grade 2 and above (see Fig. 9). A borderline (5 mm) Mantoux is equivalent to a Heaf Grade 2–3. In routine testing prior to immunization, a negative test indicates a need for BCG. A borderline result (Heaf Grade 2) means an individual is probably already immune. Those above Grade 2 require referral to a specialist to check that active disease is not present.

How given—BCG

Vaccine is reconstituted with supplied diluent and 0.05 ml (under 3 months) or 0.1 ml (all older individuals) given by intradermal injection (Fig. 8, p. 156) on the arm (customarily the left, see Fig. 7, p. 155). **A separate needle and syringe must be used for each individual and jet-injectors are not to be used.**

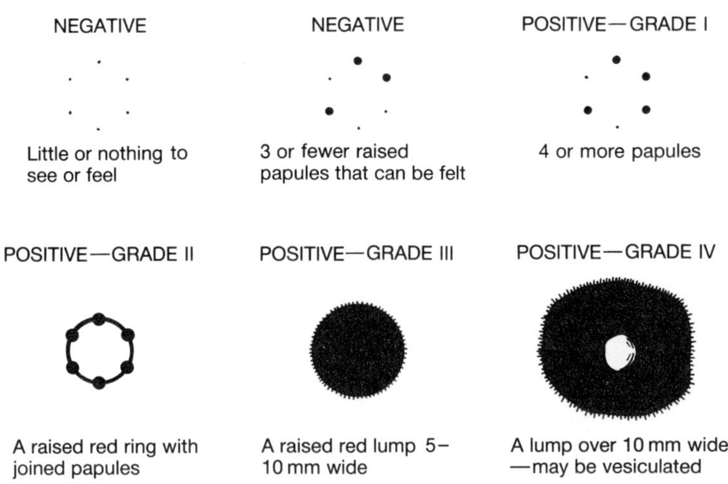

Fig. 9 Guide to reading Heaf test results.

Reactions

In most babies and children (and adults) there is a local reaction at the BCG site starting from 2–6 weeks after immunization. This begins as papules which can later discharge. No treatment is needed but parents may wish to use a dry, non-occlusive dressing. The child can still be bathed and go swimming (when a waterproof 'elastoplast' should be put on temporarily). This reaction is a local BCG infection and eventually heals leaving a small scar. More severe reactions do occur. They include prolonged deep ulceration, lymphadenitis, and osteomyelitis. **Their most common cause is faulty technique resulting in a subcutaneous rather than an intradermal injection**. Where these occur specialist advice must be sought.

Notes

1. Testing immunity after BCG

Immunity is not usually tested after immunization. A normal local reaction (see above) can be taken as indicator of success. High-risk individuals, eg health-service staff and children immunized at birth, may require sensitivity testing.

2. Skin disease

Individuals with skin disease so severe as to contraindicate BCG are extremely rare. With conditions such as eczema or psoriasis, PPD and BCG should be injected into disease-free skin.

3. Which arm?

It is customary to use the left arm (rather than the non-preferred) so that the eventual scar can be identified later.

4. Combining with other immunizations

As BCG is a live vaccine three weeks should elapse between it and any other live immunizations. In addition, immunization into the same arm should be avoided for three months as sometimes this results in painful axillary (arm-pit) lymph nodes.

Typhoid immunization

Inactivated vaccine

Immunization strategy

Protection of susceptibles.

Preparation

A monovalent vaccine of killed *Salmonella typhi*.

Effectiveness

This vaccine gives only moderate time-limited protection, lasting one year after a single dose, three years after two doses.

Indications

As the disease tends to be mild in children, and the protection afforded is only moderate, emphasis should be placed on good hygiene.

Contraindications

1. Acute febrile illness or chronic illness;
2. age under one year;
3. pregnancy.

How given

As im or deep sc injection: The intradermal route is not used for the first injection, though it can be on subsequent occasions when the dose is 0.1 ml for all.

Dosage

For children from one to nine years, each dose is 0.25 ml; for adults, 0.5 ml.

Reactions

Mild to moderate local or general reactions are common in adults, less so in children. General reactions are common. Where these are troublesome but immunization is considered necessary, the intradermal route is more likely to avoid discomfort.

Yellow fever immunization

Live vaccine

Immunization strategy

Protection of susceptibles.

Preparation

A freeze-dried preparation of live attenuated virus grown on chick embryos. This is only administered in designated yellow-fever vaccination centres and by a few general practitioners. A full list of centres is in the DH book *Immunization against infectious disease.*

Effectiveness

This is high, with immunity from a single dose lasting at least 10 years.

Indications

All children over nine months (and adults) travelling to or stopping in an endemic country. See the DH leaflet (Further reading, no. 13*a*) for a current list of countries who require a certificate. Immunization is only given in designated Yellow Fever Centres.

Contraindications

1. Acute febrile illness is a reason for deferring immunization for one week;
2. age under nine months;
3. immunodeficiency;
4. extreme hypersensitivity to neomycin or polymyxin, egg or chicken protein.
5. Pregnancy.

Reactions

Mild local or general reactions are relatively common, more severe reactions rare. Encephalitis has occurred in young infants, which is the reason for age under nine months being a contra-indication.

Immunoglobulins given to children

Immunoglobulins give immediate but short-lived (passive) immunity. The preparations used in the UK are predominantly from human sources. Concern has been expressed that they could be contaminated by HIV (human immunodeficiency virus) and so cause AIDS. The preparation process of these products, however, is such as to kill this (and all other) viruses.

Some immunoglobulins are given by deep im injection and others intravenously. Where volumes are large and the child is slim the buttock may be used (but with care to avoid the area of the sciatic nerve, see Fig. 7, p. 155).

SPECIFIC DISEASES AND IMMUNOGLOBULINS

Chickenpox

VZIG (varicella/zoster immunoglobulin). This is indicated for: immunodepressed children in contact with chickenpox or zoster (shingles); babies delivered to mothers who develop varicella in the week before or after delivery (see pp. 45–6); babies in the first month of age who are in contact with chickenpox or shingles and whose mothers have no history of chickenpox (the dose of VZIG is: 0–5 years, 250 mg; 6–10 years 500 mg; 11–14 years 750 mg; 15 years upwards 1000 g).

Measles

Human normal immunoglobulin (HNIG) given to immunodepressed children (see p. 219) exposed to measles. The dosage is 250 mg for babies under 12 months; 500 mg for those aged 1–2 years; and 750 mg for those over two years. A preparation of concentrated human measles immunoglobulin is available in Scotland.

Mumps

No specific immunoglobulin is now given or available. Immunodepressed children may be considered for normal immunoglobulin if exposed to mumps.

Hepatitis A

See p. 165.

Hepatitis B

Immunoglobulin is indicated along with hepatitis B vaccination (see p. 168) for infants of high-risk carrier mothers (those HBeAg positive or both HBeAg and anti-HBe negative). It is also given to infants whose mothers suffered acute hepatitis B in the last trimester of pregnancy or early in the postnatal period. The dosage is a single 5.0 ml (500 mg) intramuscular injection. The appropriate immunoglobulin is available from the Hepatitis Epidemiology Unit, Central PHLS (see p. 268) and may be repeated at monthly intervals if active immunization is delayed.

Rabies

See p. 236.

Rubella in pregnant contacts

Normal immunoglobulin is sometimes given to pregnant contacts of rubella but is of little value.

Tetanus

Tetanus specific human immunoglobulin (Humotet) is occasionally given to severely injured under-immunized children. The dosage is 250 iu (1 ml).

Practical immunization: Questions and answers

Practical immunization: questions and answers

How to use this section

This section is designed to give individual answers to many of the simple problems encountered in day-to-day immunization practice. Nurses and doctors engaged in such work will find it useful to read through the section completely. However, each question is written so that it can be read individually and hence there is a degree of repetition in the text. Readers should be aware that though in most cases the correct answer to a specific problem is to offer all indicated immunizations, there are many parents, doctors, and nurses who have been misinformed and will believe the contrary. The information and opinions they have been given are examples of **immunization myths**, for a full list of which see p. 146.

Counselling parents

In many of the situations described, parents will be seeking guidance from professionals. Families require different degrees of counselling and the nurse advising parents will need to judge which parents are particularly confused by the myths or have other concerns which are best discussed with a well-informed doctor. General practitioners and community children's doctors may occasionally have to consult community or hospital paediatricians or other specialists. Whenever possible this should be by telephone so as not to delay immunization. **It is never justifiable to deny a child protection out of ignorance**. The practice of giving diphtheria/tetanus alone and 'we'll check about pertussis' must not be undertaken. Experience is that children do not catch up later with pertussis vaccination; whooping cough catches up with them.

Homeopathy and Immunization

The council of the faculty of homeopathy strongly supports the vaccination programme and has stated that vaccination should be carried out in the normal way using the conventional tested and approved vaccines, in the absence of medical contraindications.

If a homeopath has advised against immunization in the absence of contraindications, it is likely that he is not a member of the faculty of homeopathy. When this occurs, the parents should be advised to consult a faculty member.

EARLY PROBLEMS

Difficult birth, perinatal problems, extended period in special care but no suspected brain damage

Most babies who have had difficult deliveries or a stormy period after birth should receive pertussis immunization but the doctor may need to be consulted. The recommendations for whooping cough immunization (p. 178) no longer exclude babies with a history of cerebral irritation in the neonatal period. If the baby seems to be developing normally at the time immunizations are due, pertussis should be given.

Suspected cerebral damage

If the baby is developing normally, pertussis should be given. If there is any substantial doubt over whether the child has sustained damage, **the nurse or doctor should seek advice from a paediatrician or other appropriate specialist (preferably by telephone) rather than deny the child protection against whooping cough or any other disease**.

It is often difficult to decide whether cerebral damage has taken place in babies whose stay in hospital following birth has been long and difficult. Some special-care baby units specify in their discharge summaries the immunizations that should be given. This practice is to be encouraged as not only is it helpful for primary-care staff, but also at the time first immunizations are due many families will still be attending hospital and will therefore pay close attention to the opinion of their hospital specialist. Where there is any doubt, neonatal units should give guidance over the phone to an enquiring doctor.

Documented cerebral damage

Documented cerebral damage is **not** a contraindication to pertussis immunization, and children with stable neurological conditions should be immunized with all indicated vaccines, including pertussis and MMR. Children who have suffered in the birth period also often have chronic lung disease (bronchopulmonary dysplasia) and hence are at particular risk from whooping cough. Individual evaluation is required while the nature of the damage becomes clear. **When the nurse or doctor is unsure as to whether or not to give pertussis vaccine they should seek advice from a paediatrician (preferably by telephone) rather than deny the child protection.**

Premature babies—when should immunization start?

Immunizations start two months after birth no matter how premature the baby. All the evidence points to protection being just as effective as in the term infant. Some babies will require immunization before they are discharged from neonatal units. Oral polio vaccine should not be given to resident infants. When this is done the local immunization record holders must be informed.

Small babies

Immunizations start at two months after birth irrespective of weight or gestation. The smaller the baby or child the more they are at risk if whooping cough is caught.

Breastfeeding babies

Breastfeeding does not interfere with immunization (this includes polio drops). The same is true no matter what medication the mother is taking.

Babies and children with minor illnesses

Unwell babies and children

It is important to assess each case individually and particularly to ask about feeding and to take the temperature. If the illness is minimal or in the recovery phase, the child is feeding normally, and the temperature is under 37.5°C, immunization should proceed. If the parents feel their child is just starting an illness, it will be wiser to defer immunization for a week. The same applies for babies or children who are clearly unwell in the doctor's view. A useful rule is that children should not be immunized if their axillary temperature is over 37.5°C and ill babies and children may need to be seen by a doctor for treatment of their illness. If in doubt, a medical opinion should be sought to ascertain fitness for immunization. One further useful rule used by nurses is that any baby or child whose immunizations have to be deferred on two successive weeks should see a doctor at, or as soon as possible after, the second occasion.

Babies who are snuffly or chesty

Some babies always seem to be a bit snuffly or chesty and others carry on coughing long after a respiratory illness. If the baby is apyrexial and feeding well, it is safe to ignore chronic snuffles, coughs, and wheezes, and proceed with immunization; otherwise such babies would never receive protection. Any child whose immunization is deferred on two successive weeks should be seen by a doctor.

Babies and children with a rash

As long as the baby or child is well and has no fever she can be immunized.

Babies and children who have had contact with an infectious illness recently

As long as the baby or child is well he can be immunized. This is particularly important for measles where a dose of MMR protects unimmunized children from the worst effects of the illness.

Babies and children with diarrhoea

If a baby or child is generally unwell with acute diarrhoea then all immunizations should be deferred for a week. In the essentially well individual, diarrhoea is irrelevant to all injected immunizations and these should all be given. However, polio drops should be delayed unless there is substantial doubt whether the family will return, in which case a better strategy is to give the drops plus an extra dose at a later date. Some babies and children always have loose stools (toddler diarrhoea) and if such a child is well, give polio drops.

Babies and children reported to have already had an illness

Usually this is when the baby is supposed to have already had measles or whooping cough. Nurses should never tell parents that immunization will not be needed but must first consult the doctor. Many babies who are reported to have had measles (which is rare in the UK before the first birthday) or whooping cough have, in fact, had another illness with some resemblance to the rash of measles or the cough of whooping cough. Measles in particular is over-diagnosed: almost any rash will eventually be called measles if it is presented to enough people! Babies and children who are not immunized for this reason will probably catch the real illness later, and this is the principal way they may seem to have a disease twice. Even if they have actually had the illness, there is no extra risk from being immunized. Only positive serology is acceptable proof of measles infection and is not recommended and then the child must still have MMR to receive protection against mumps and rubella. A positive immunofluorescence test or culture of *Bordetella* is the only acceptable proof of *B. pertussis* infection. Girls with an alleged history of rubella should still be immunized in secondary school unless serology shows the girl to be immune. See also Parental counselling, p. 151.

Babies and children on antibiotics and other medicines

Babies and children on antibiotics

As long as they have almost recovered from their illness, it is acceptable to proceed with immunization. A nurse or community children's doctor may decide to first consult the GP who prescribed the medicine. Immunization works perfectly well and is just as safe for children on antibiotics.

Babies or children on other common medicines, e.g. nystatin elixir

Babies and children may be immunized as long as they are well.

Children and babies having steroids

This is only relevant for live vaccines (polio, MMR, BCG, and rubella—see list p. 218) and even then only in the rare circumstances where high doses of steroids are being given. The criteria are a course of injected or oral steroids of 2 mg/kg or more for over one continuous week in the preceding three months. Shorter courses, lower doses, and locally acting preparations (e.g. inhaled Becotide and topical skin steroids) do not interfere with immunization.

Previous reactions

Babies and children who have had a previous severe reaction to a vaccine which included pertussis

If the next indicated immunization contains pertussis, check whether the reaction meets the criteria given. The definition of a severe reaction is:

Local: An extensive area of redness at the vaccination site which becomes indurated (hard) and involves most of the front and side of the thigh, or a major part of the circumference of the upper arm.

General: Fever over 39.5°C occurring within 48 hours, or any one of the following occurring within 72 hours, of an immunization: anaphylaxis, bronchospasm (wheeze), laryngeal oedema, generalized collapse, prolonged unresponsiveness, convulsions, prolonged inconsolable screaming.

On the uncommon occasion where the reaction meets these criteria pertussis should be excluded from future injections. This must be documented and the reaction recorded and reported (see p. 159).

Where parents have experienced less severe reactions in their child they may find counselling from a well-informed doctor useful. Where a reaction has been less than that described, or the immunizing nurse or doctor is unsure whether it fits the criteria, they should never advise immunizing with just diphtheria and tetanus. They should seek advice from a paediatrician or other appropriate specialist (preferably by phone) rather than deny the child protection. See also Parental Counselling, p. 151.

Children who have had a previous reaction to a vaccine which did not include pertussis

Rarely the second or third injection containing tetanus and diphtheria vaccine (pertussis omitted because of a reaction following the previous dose) also results in a reaction. Skin tests do not help in determining which vaccine is the cause of the reaction. It is recommended that tetanus is given alone following a clear-explanation to the parents that there is a risk of reaction, unless there has been an anaphylactic response previously in which case no further immunization with tetanus or diphtheria vaccine is recommended.

Fits, febrile convulsions, developmental delay, neurological disease, cerebral palsy

Babies and children who have had fits or febrile convulsions

Parents may call temper tantrums, breath-holding attacks, rigors, or faints 'fits'. There are also many different kinds of fits, some more relevant to immunization than others (see next paragraph). A personal history of fits is no longer a contraindication to pertussis immunization, and children with stable neurological conditions, such as epilepsy, may be vaccinated (see p. 178). Hence most babies or children who have had fits can be immunized with pertussis vaccine. Parents of such children are usually anxious about immunization and these are circumstances where cases require individual evaluation by the doctor with the parents. Fits are no reason for denying a child MMR, but precautions may be needed to prevent or deal with any febrile reactions (see p. 175). Parents whose child has had a febrile convulsion need reminding that their child is especially likely to have another if it catches measles and so immunization with MMR is especially important. Fits are not relevant to other immunizations. If the family is being cared for by a paediatrician it will be wise to agree on a joint community/hospital immunization policy.

Babies and children who had **neonatal fits** due to hypocalcaemia can certainly be immunized with pertussis vaccine. The same applies for children whose fits were due to hypoglycaemia or hypoxia.

Babies and children with mild developmental delay

All immunizations including pertussis and MMR may be given. It is important that the parents understand about their child's delay before immunization commences.

Babies and children with serious developmental delay

Most children with severe developmental delay should not be denied protection, including that of pertussis and MMR vaccine. If the condition is stable (e.g. in established cerebral palsy), then immunization should be given. Other cases will, however, need assessment, and where a paediatrician is already involved she or he should be contacted first. This particularly applies if the underlying cause of the delay is undiagnosed. Such assessment is best anticipated prior to any immunization being due.

Neurological disease

Most of these children will be under the care of a paediatrician who should be consulted. For progressive cerebral disease, such as neuro-degenerative conditions (**but not muscular dystrophy**) and other neurological disorders such as tuberous sclerosis, it may be reasonable to omit pertussis, while polio, diphtheria, tetanus, and MMR vaccines should be given as usual (see also next paragraph).

Stable neurological conditions (cerebral palsy, spina bifida, hydrocephalus, etc.)

The child should be given pertussis immunization as well as all other indicated vaccines (taking precautions for MMR if the child has had fits). It will be advisable to contact the child's paediatrician prior to immunization to ensure a consistent policy.

Non-neurological illness

The baby or child with long-term chest or heart condition (eg cystic fibrosis or congenital heart disease)

It is particularly important that these children are protected with pertussis and MMR. When the child is chronically or usually unwell (e.g. the cyanotic child) immunization must not be put off without consulting the doctor. The latter will need to bear in mind that to prevent deterioration of their condition as a result of whooping cough or measles such children may need to be immunized when in a state of chronic ill health. Children with cystic fibrosis may benefit from regular influenza immunization. Parents should be advised to contact their doctors to arrange urgent immunization as early as possible during an influenza epidemic.

Immunodeficient children

See p. 218.

Down's syndrome, simple mental retardation

As for stable neurological conditions, these children are entitled to all the usual immunizations. Some children with Down's seem especially vulnerable to respiratory infections and are constantly snuffly or chesty, and this is not a contraindication to immunization.

Babies and children with asthma, eczema, hay fever, or simple allergies

All routine immunizations should be given, including whooping cough and MMR.

The child with extreme or severe egg allergy

For MMR or monovalent measles this is only important in the extremely rare circumstances when there is a history of anaphylaxis, in which case further advice should be sought prior to immunization with these vaccines. The same applies for influenza and yellow fever vaccines. All other routine protection should be given and the commoner forms of egg allergy (diarrhoea, skin rashes) are of no importance. There is no value in intradermal skin testing with MMR vaccine in children with a documented history of egg allergy.

FAMILY HISTORY

First degree relatives have had fits

These children should have all immunizations, including whooping cough and MMR. If the fits are due to idiopathic epilepsy, a doctor should counsel the parents concerning management of the child after immunization as there is a very small additional risk of a febrile convulsion (see MMR, p. 175).
See also Parental Counselling, pp. 151–2.

Grandparents, aunts, uncles, fifth cousins, etc. having fits

Any fits in relatives beyond the immediate (first-degree) family are irrelevant to immunization. The child can receive all immunizations without special precautions.

A brother or sister had a severe immunization reaction

All immunizations should be given; however, parents may understandably be nervous and may need to consult the doctor before proceeding. See also Parental counselling, p. 151.

Family history of asthma, eczema, hay fever, or allergies

These are all irrelevant to immunization. The baby or child should be given full protection.

Administrative problems

Interrupted immunization course

In this case the immunizer should give the next immunization that the child is due to receive. If more than one is overdue (for example Triple, polio, and MMR), then all should be given at the same session. However, if more than one Triple is overdue they still need to be spaced apart at the usual intervals.
It is never necessary to restart an immunization course.

Pre-school booster—prior injections overdue

When children come for their pre-school booster it often turns out that they have missed out on some immunizations. Children should catch up with these on this occasion. A classical story is a child who presents at booster time having only had two Triples (DTP) and polios. She or he should have the third Triple, the MMR, and polio at one visit. They will then need the diphtheria/tetanus and polio boosters in three years' time. **If only the measles has been missed, the pre-school booster is given at the usual time with the MMR in the other arm.**

Pre-school booster—measles already given

The child should be given MMR as well as the diphtheria/tetanus and polio booster.

Older children behind in immunization

If over three but under 10 years old, the child should have any immunizations missed including MMR (up to the sixteenth birthday). This includes pertussis as this child will place any younger children (especially babies) at risk if he or she catches whooping cough.

If over 10 years old, the child should have any immunizations that have been missed. If diphtheria is needed, the special adult vaccine is required; alternatively a one-fifth dose (0.1 ml) of the normal vaccine can be given. There is no need for a Schick test (a measurement of immunity to diphtheria). It is important to remember to ask if the child has already had a tetanus injection at casualty or from a general practitioner.

Giving two immunizations at once

It is acceptable to give MMR, and diphtheria, tetanus, pertussis, and polio vaccine simultaneously, but 3 weeks should elapse between BCG and other live vaccines such as MMR. **However, it is important never to mix vaccines in the same syringe**. If giving two injections, it is good practice to give one in each arm and to document this so that it is possible to attribute any local reaction to the correct vaccine.

Once live vaccine has been given it is usually recommended to wait three weeks before giving another. However, the evidence that this is of any clinical importance is weak, and where two live vaccines are inadvertently given within the time period it is not justified to repeat either. When BCG is given it is recommended to allow three months to elapse before giving any other vaccination in the same arm, as this has been associated with painful axillary lymph node swelling.

Child due for routine immunization who has recently had a tetanus injection

It is simplest to ignore the tetanus and proceed with the indicated immunization.

Children of pregnant mothers

All immunizations should be given, including polio.

Recent immigrants

It can be difficult to find out what immunizations have been given to immigrants, and it may be necessary to treat the children and the rest of the family as if they were unimmunized and start a complete programme (see p. 266 for schedules). It is particularly important to check the rubella serology of any young women in the family and to give rubella vaccine if necessary. A Heaf or Mantoux test is always needed if the family has come from an area with high levels of tuberculosis (India, Bangladesh, Pakistan, East Asia, Africa, and other Third World countries).

Non-English speaking parents

An interpreter is mandatory for taking a history. Simply obtaining a signature without proper counselling is bad practice.

Children from another area with inadequate records

To wait for full details from another district can mean an intolerable delay and such children should not be denied protection. It is wise to involve a doctor in deciding on immunization, not least as the children may have other medical or developmental problems needing assessment and treatment.

Unknown family history, fostered or adopted babies and children

While efforts should be made to obtain a family history, it is worth noting that only fits in parents or siblings are relevant. When the history is unobtainable, the case should be considered by a doctor. The chances of the child catching measles or whooping cough are high and therefore the risks arising from leaving the child unprotected are considerably higher than from any immunization. A family history is often deficient in fostered and adopted children. In these cases immunization must not be delayed and should proceed normally.

Children in care

Written permission has to be given by the appropriate member of the Social Services Department for children to enter a course of immunizations. Care needs to be taken in getting a reliable history concerning previous immunizations and any severe reaction. Social services should be asked to provide such information at the time of immunization.

Wards of court

Written permission will need to be sought from the Court. This can take months and should be thought about well before immunizations are due. As for children in care, a reliable history concerning previous immunizations should be obtained if at all possible.

Mothers under 16

The mother is usually the person to give any written consent. Special care should be taken to ensure counselling is adequate.

Person accompanying the baby or child scarcely knows them

It should be parents or guardians who give any necessary written consent for entering an immunization programme. For subsequent injections the person who brings the child needs to know him well enough to give a proper history about reactions to previous immunizations.

OTHER PROBLEMS

Babies who vomit after polio drops

This is only important if the baby has a substantial vomit in the first hour after immunization, in which case more drops should be given.

Blood transfusion

A child who has recently had a transfusion can be immunized. It is unusual for children to need transfusions and it will be sensible to ask the reason for this so as to check that the child does not have an immunodeficient state (e.g. leukaemia) that necessitated the transfusion. It is suggested that blood transfusion may interfere with rubella immunization. This eventuality most commonly arises in the postnatal seronegative woman who had a transfusion and needs immunization.

General anaesthetic

Any child may have a mild reaction to an immunization and this could complicate an anaesthetic. Hence immunization should be avoided in the three days (12 days for MMR) before an anaesthetic for a pre-arranged operation. Children can have any immunization needed as soon as they are over an anaesthetic, and there is no reason to believe any anaesthetic reduces the effectiveness of immunization. There is no reason for putting off routine surgery outside of these time limits and an urgently needed operation should proceed irrespective of recent immunizations.

After injury

Severe injuries

Burns or wounds with the following features require emergency treatment, including consideration for protection against tetanus: a significant amount of dead tissue; or a puncture-type wound; or soiling with earth or other material likely to be contaminated with tetanus; or obvious evidence of infection; or any wound where there has been more than six hours before receiving surgical treatment; or a human or animal bite.

The wound should be cleaned and the child given anti-tetanus protection according to the following schedule.

1. **Children (or adults) not known to have completed a full course of tetanus injections** (the number of tetanus injections will depend on the age of the child: a one-year-old should have had three injections, a five-year-old four injections, etc.) and **children (or adults) who had their last tetanus injection more than 10 years previously** should all have anti-tetanus immunoglobulin by intramuscular injection in one limb and the first of a course of three tetanus injections in the other limb. The remaining tetanus injections are given at monthly intervals or (for the child under three years of age) as per the national schedule.

2. **Children (or adults) who have only had a single injection** should be treated as (1) with anti-tetanus immunoglobulin and an immediate tetanus injection but they will only need one more tetanus injection later.

3. **Children (or adults) who completed a primary course (three injections) or had a booster within the previous 10 years** do not require immunoglobulin, and only need a single tetanus injection, tetanus vaccine if the risk of infection is high, as might follow contamination with manure.

Less severe injuries

If the wound is less severe than listed above, a child midway through a primary immunization course does not need a booster (for example, a nine-month-old with a minor scratch who has had two DTP immunizations). Some doctors may prefer to give a tetanus toxoid injection in casualty, especially if only one immunization has been given. If this is done, the local health authority and the child's general practitioner must be notified.

Immunization and protection of infants and children with specific problems

Many of the children covered below will be under the care of both hospital specialists and general practitioners. Early consultation is recommended to ensure agreement on immunization policy. Nothing is more confusing for parents than to receive differing advice and if this occurs the child is usually denied protection. When a normal immunization schedule is recommended this is as per the national schedule (on back cover).

Practical immunization: questions and answersImmunization: children with specific problems **Achondroplasia/hypochondroplasia**—normal immunization schedule.

AIDS—see HIV infection (p. 217).

Allergy—a history of allergy eczema or asthma is not a contraindication to immunization. When there has been an anaphylactic response to eggs, MMR (measles/mumps/rubella), influenza, and yellow fever vaccines should not be given without specialist advice.

Asplenia—pneumococcal vaccine is recommended in addition to normal schedules. Vaccine alone will not give complete protection against pneumococcal disease, particularly in children with sickle-cell disease where extra protection with oral penicillin is necessary. Penicillin is recommended for children following splenectomy.

Arthritis—see juvenile rheumatoid arthritis.

Asthma—normal immunization schedule. If very severe, consider influenza immunization.

Birth asphyxia—normal schedule in absence of fits or developmental delay. Infants with early neonatal fits following asphyxia come into the 'problem history' group (see p. 178) for pertussis. The presence of bronchopulmonary dysplasia/chronic lung disease is a strong indication for pertussis immunization.

Cerebral palsy—normal schedule if stable; if history of seizures, advise on temperature control (see p. 178).

Congenital heart disease—normal immunization schedule. Consider influenza immunization for children with cyanotic heart disease over six months of age. See also endocarditis prophylaxis, p. 220.

Cystic fibrosis—normal immunization schedule. Annual influenza vaccination is recommended in children over six months.

Diabetes mellitus—normal immunization schedule.

Down's syndrome—normal immunization schedule.

Endocarditis prophylaxis—see p. 220.

Endocrine disorders—normal immunization schedule.

Epilepsy—see febrile convulsions.

Febrile convulsions—pertussis immunization is normally completed before these develop. However, where they have occurred, or immunization has been delayed, pertussis vaccine should be given (see p. 178) as well as MMR. Immunoglobulin should **not** be used and parents should be advised on temperature control.

Growth hormone deficiency—normal immunization schedule.

Haemophilia and other non-malignant bleeding problems—normal immunization schedule. Give all injections subcutaneously (or intradermally if indicated) **not** intramuscularly.

Heart disease—see congenital heart disease above.

Human immunodeficiency virus (HIV)—These children are likely to be under the care of a specialist who should be consulted for discussion of an appropriate immunization course.

1. HIV-positive but asymptomatic children, including those of indeterminate status (HIV-positive children under 15 months where the reason for positivity may be passive transfer of maternal antibody), should receive the normal immunization schedule including: polio, diphtheria, pertussis, tetanus, MMR/measles, rubella. BCG should **not** be given. Inactivated polio (IPV) may be given to a child when there is the risk of a parent being immunodepressed.

2. Symptomatic HIV-positive children, can receive live virus vaccines (except BCG) as the benefits of protection outweigh the risks from the vaccines, especially where the diseases against which the children are being protected are prevalent. They should receive all appropriate inactivated vaccines.

Hydrocephalus—normal immunization schedule. In the presence of fits special consideration for pertussis immunization should be given (see p. 178) and MMR (see p. 175).

Immunodeficient/Immunodepressed—This state may follow disease or treatment. The following groups of children should not receive live vaccines (p. 143). For HIV infection see p. 217.

(1) patients receiving immunosuppressive treatment including general irradiation; those suffering from malignant conditions such as lymphoma, leukaemia, Hodgkin's disease, or other tumours of the reticuloendothelial system; patients with impaired immunological mechanism as, for example, in hypogammaglobulinaemia;

(2) children with immunosuppression from disease or therapy (eg in remission from acute leukaemia) until at least six months after chemotherapy has finished;

(3) children treated with systemic corticosteroids at high dose (2 mg/kg/day for more than a week) until at least three months after treatment has stopped (children on lower daily doses of systemic corticosteroids for less than two weeks, and those who have moved onto either continuously lower doses or alternate day regimens for longer periods, may be given live virus vaccines).

All inactivated vaccines may be given to immunodepressed children, but they may not be as effective.

The close contacts (siblings, class-mates, close friends) of immunosupressed children **must** be immunized with MMR. Measles has killed many immunodepressed children. **Community paediatricians and nurses bear a special responsibility to see that MMR uptake is particularly high in any school or day-care facility where such children are placed.** There is no risk of virus transmission following measles, mumps, or rubella vaccines. Oral poliomyelitis vaccine (OPV) should not be given to these children, their siblings or other household contacts; inactivated vaccine (IPV) should be used in its place. In the case of malignancies, a complete immunization history is needed at the time of diagnosis and historical and serological evidence sought for immunity to measles, chickenpox, and rubella. Where either suggest non-immunity, children in categories (1) and (2) above will need an injection of immunoglobulin as soon as possible after exposure to measles or chickenpox. The specialist team looking after them must be contacted **immediately** such exposure is suspected. Children with congenital immune deficiencies may not respond to vaccines and some need regular doses of immunoglobulin. Children who develop chickenpox should be treated with acyclovir, as soon as the signs appear. Post-vaccination immunity may be lost following treatment with immunosuppressive drugs. For this reason, it may be appropriate to reimmunize children after such treatment. Live vaccine can be reintroduced 6–12 months after treatment has been completed.

Juvenile rheumatoid arthritis—check rubella serology in girls and if negative immunize; delay if in active stage of disease.

Leukaemia—see immunodepressed.

Malabsorption—normal immunization schedule including oral polio.

Malignancies—see immunodepressed.

Meningitis—normal immunization schedule.

Metabolic disorders—many may receive the normal immunization schedule. This is, however, such a range of disorders, with some children in delicate metabolic states, that individual cases should be discussed with their supervising doctor.

Muscular dystrophy—normal immunization schedule.

Nephrotic syndrome—require pneumovax. Immunoglobulin if exposed to varicella and measles.

Pregnancy—live vaccines are to be avoided unless the risk is high. Examples are women travelling to areas where polio or yellow fever is endemic. Inadvertent rubella immunization is not an indication for termination.

Prematurity—normal schedule for all immunizations given at appropriate times from birth.

Sickle-cell disease—see asplenia.

Spina bifida—normal immunization schedule.

Splenectomy—see asplenia.

Steroids—see immunodepressed.

Thalassaemia—see asplenia.

Toddler diarrhoea—normal immunization schedule, including oral polio.

Tonsillectomy, adenoidectomy, etc.—normal immunization schedule, including oral polio.

Turner's syndrome—normal immunization schedule.

ENDOCARDITIS PROPHYLAXIS FOR CHILDREN WITH HEART DEFECTS

Children with congenital heart defects are at risk from bacterial endocarditis caused by the transient bacteraemia released by certain dental and surgical procedures involving mucosa and infected tissue. They should be protected by antibiotic prophylaxis.

At particular risk are children with prosthetic heart valves or systemic to pulmonary artery shunts, but bacterial endocarditis should be considered when any child with a heart abnormality develops an unexplained febrile illness, especially if it follows a dental or surgical operation.

Parents should be told about the importance of high standards of oral hygiene and regular dental inspections for their children. It is helpful if they can be given brief written instructions about antibiotic prophylaxis to which they can refer when necessary or draw to the attention of dentists and surgeons at the appropriate times.

Prophylaxis should continue after the surgical repair of most heart defects but for a few the risk of endocarditis is so small that antibiotics are not recommended. These include: (a) repaired ostium secundium atrial septal defects (after six months); (b) closed patent ductus arteriosus.

For general dental treatment likely to cause gum bleeding, especially for extractions

The following should be given one hour before the procedure: amoxycillin 3.0 g orally to children over 10 years, and 1.5 g orally to children under 10; or, if there is an allergy to penicillin, erythromycin 1.0 g orally to children over 10 years and 0.5 g orally to children under 10. Note: these doses are 'rounded off' for convenience to suit children of school age likely to need dental treatment without general anaesthesia.

For procedures in hospital with a general anaesthetic

The following should be given intravenously with induction of anaesthesia:

1. Dental and respiratory tract surgery: amoxycillin 50 mg/kg.
2. Gastrointestinal and genitourinary surgery: amoxycillin 50 mg/kg plus gentamicin 2 mg/kg. Note: if there is penicillin allergy, replace amoxycillin with erythromicin 20 mg/kg (as lactobionate) given slowly.
3. Children with prosthetic heart valves (at special risk): gentamicin 2 mg/kg plus vancomycin 20 mg/kg given slowly.

Travel abroad

Travel abroad

International travel is increasing: in 1979 UK residents made 14 million trips abroad; by 1986 the figure was 23 million, 12 per cent to destinations beyond Europe.

Most children travelling abroad fall into one of two major groups: (a) those taking a holiday in Europe and the Mediterranean; and (b) those returning with their parents to the countries of origin, of which the Indian subcontinent (ISC) is the most common, followed by West Africa. In addition, smaller numbers undertake more ambitious trips and travel advice may be needed for children visiting almost any country in the world.

The infections to which a child may be exposed include those commoner in less developed countries, many of which are amenable to immunization or chemoprophylaxis (eg typhoid, polio, diphtheria, yellow fever, malaria) and also those which remain prevalent in Britain (gastroenteritis, whooping cough, hepatitis, measles, tuberculosis). With air travel, almost all diseases contracted abroad may be incubating on return. Hence, a history of recent travel must be sought in any child with fever, gastrointestinal, or other symptoms suggestive of infection.

Health advice for travel is a complex subject and a text can never be up to date. Also, the protection recommended for an extended stay may be very different from that for a holiday. This section simply outlines the advice most commonly sought and lists the sources which the health-care worker or traveller can consult for more detailed and current information (see also Further reading, p. 271.)

General advice

Travel abroad has many potential hazards, not all associated with infection. These include different safety standards, exposure to extremes of climate, and language difficulties all compounding ignorance of the local medical system. To a certain extent, parents must exercise their own common sense regarding their child's visit. A family checklist is: appropriate clothing, entertainment for the journey, adequate protection against sunburn, medical insurance, immunization prophylaxis, and simple medications.

These topics are well covered in many popular and professional publications, two examples of which are listed in Further reading nos 11 and 12 (p. 272). Specific guidelines for individual countries are also provided in the DH leaflet *The Travellers Guide to Health* (Further reading, no. 13*a* Appendix 6) which is updated annually and available on Prestel, page 50063.

Simple precautions

Eighty per cent of holiday-acquired infections (mostly the various forms of gastroenteritis) are water and/or food borne, and though they are not preventable by immunization, simple precautions will help to protect all family members. Some guidelines are given below. The extent to which they are followed will depend on local conditions and family preference. However, it is wise to emphasize to parents that diarrhoea is a common cause of a spoilt holiday and may be a serious risk.

1. Scrupulous attention to hand hygiene especially after using the toilet, nappy-changing, and before meals. Soap and/or toilet paper may be unavailable locally.

2. Where the water supply may be of uncertain quality (that is most countries outside northern Europe, North America, New Zealand, Australia, and urban South Africa), the traveller should not drink water from taps or other sources. Hot, bottled, or canned drinks with well-known brand names are safest. Alternatively, water can be treated. If visible matter is present, the water should first be strained through a closely woven cloth. Sterilization is achieved by boiling for five minutes or disinfecting. Appropriate disinfectants are chlorine and iodine (either liquid bleach, tincture of iodine, or 'sterilizing' tablets). Iodine is preferable as chlorine is less effective. All tablets have makers' instructions. Tincture of iodine (2 per cent) should be used at a concentration of 4 drops to 1 litre of water; the water is then allowed to stand for 30 minutes before use.

3. In the same countries as those where water precautions are advised the following should be avoided: raw vegetables, salads, unpeeled fruit, raw shellfish, cream, ice-cream, underdone meat or fish, uncooked or cold pre-cooked food, and ice

cubes. Similarly, unpasteurized milk (unless boiled) and cheese apart from that known to be made from pasteurized milk, may also carry infection.

4. Self-caterers should cook meat well. Fruit and vegetables should be washed thoroughly in clean soapy water. If they are not then being cooked, they should be soaked for half an hour in treated water at three times the concentration of disinfectant used for purifying drinking water (see above).
5. In case a child develops gastroenteritis, the family need to pack some oral rehydration mixture (eg Dioralyte, Rehidrat). One cupful for each loose stool is a memorable dosage but parents must seek medical help if excessive vomiting, severe diarrhoea, drowsiness, or other signs of dehydration occur, especially in a young baby (see p. 58).
6. Children (and adults) should not play on beaches or swim in water visibly polluted with sewage.

SPECIFIC ADVICE FOR PARTICULAR COUNTRIES AND DISEASES

Information sources

Because the specific advice can change so frequently, it is best for the traveller or the professional either to consult regularly updated publications or to contact designated information centres. The former are: the DH pamphlet *Travellers Guide to Health* (T1), (Further reading, no. 13*a* Appendix 6); the WHO booklet *Vaccination certificate requirements and health advice for international travel* (Further reading, no. 14); the medical newspaper *Pulse* (table updated monthly), MIMS, and the DoH publication, *Travel information for medical practitioners* (Further reading, no 13*b*). These list the advice and requirements by country. However, the advice is not always consistent. Requirements tend to lag behind the times (until recently a few countries still needed proof of smallpox immunization!) and protection in addition to the formal requirements is frequently advisable. Also, what is necessary for a brief trip to a country's main city may be very different from the protection appropriate for an extended stay up-country. The main information centres are listed in Appendix 5 (p. 268) and a more detailed list of specialist associations is provided in *Travellers' health* (Further reading, no. 11).

Parents taking children on a complicated tour or extended trip may find the Medical Advisory Services for Travellers Abroad (MASTA) useful. Based at the London School of Hygiene and Tropical Medicine, it tailors a personalized health brief to the specific journey and medical history (see Appendix 5, p. 268 for address). It does charge a fee. Family application forms are available from MASTA and most branches of Boots.

Routine immunizations for travel

Polio

There have recently been several cases of poliomyelitis in the children of African and Asian immigrant parents. Although born in Britain, they had either not started or completed their immunization before being taken on visits to the home country. It cannot be assumed that a course will be completed abroad. The vaccine may not be available, and some parents do not realize the need for continuing the course. Such high-risk babies must be fully protected before they leave, by starting in the neonatal period if necessary. It is equally important to advise that children of any age visiting an endemic area (for practical purposes all less developed countries) should be fully immunized against polio. Adults accompanying them should have boosters if they have had none in the preceding 10 years.

Diphtheria, measles

Both are common in the ISC and Africa. All British children should be protected by ensuring immunization is up to date. No booster will be needed for fully immunized children or adults. Children going to the USA and entering school or registered day-care will be required by law to produce documentary proof of immunization, including MMR.

Tuberculosis

Children at risk are those making extended visits to developing countries. If the child has not had BCG as a neonate, it must be given before visiting an endemic area for a month or more. Forward planning is needed as a Heaf or Mantoux test must be used first and six weeks should elapse between BCG and departure.

Tetanus

Whatever and wherever the holiday, the consultation for advice should include ensuring up-to-date tetanus vaccination (NB: not more frequently than 10-yearly after the primary course).

ADDITIONAL IMMUNIZATIONS AND CHEMOPROPHYLAXIS COMMONLY RECOMMENDED FOR TRAVEL

Typhoid

There are between 50 and 60 notifications of typhoid in children each year in England and Wales, the majority acquired overseas, chiefly in the ISC. Prevention is most effectively achieved by good standards of personal hygiene and avoidance of contaminated food and water. A vaccine is available but is only moderately protective and its effectiveness wanes rapidly (see p. 194).

Cholera

This disease is endemic in the ISC with epidemics in Africa, the Middle East, and occasionally the Mediterranean. A handful of cases occur annually in the UK, all acquired abroad. As for typhoid, good hygiene is the best prevention and the vaccine is of very limited effectiveness (see p. 194).

Yellow fever

This disease occurs in two endemic zones, Central Africa and the northern zone of South America, with cases occurring in both urban and rural settings. Cases are almost unheard of in Britain but travellers to these countries are certainly at risk and must be protected. In addition, many countries require the immunization which is used in two situations: (a) for travellers to the endemic zones; and (b) for travellers to non-endemic areas which require evidence of immunity from visitors who have passed through an endemic zone *en route* (these countries have climates and mosquitoes which would favour transmission, hence they wish to prevent disease introduction). See *Protect your health abroad* (Further reading, no. 13*a* Appendix 6) for a current list of the centres offering immunization. For a description of the disease, see p. 131; and of the immunization, see p. 195.

Malaria

(See also p. 83.) In 1986 British families made 1.2 million trips to endemic areas: Africa, including the Mediterranean coast; the Indian subcontinent; the tropical Far East; South and Central America, plus Haiti. Asian or African parents are often unaware of the need for chemoprophylaxis and, consequently, now make up half the cases reported in the UK. Often their home area was relatively free from malaria when they lived there, or they may believe that their childhood immunity should still protect them. The latter is certainly untrue, and families must be persuaded of the importance of prevention. There are three approaches to prevention of malaria and travel advice must include **all** of these.

Avoidance of mosquito bites

These are most likely after sunset and indoors.

1. It is recommended to sleep under a mosquito net (available from MASTA (see Appendix 5, p. 270); nets are priced £25–32), preferably one impregnated with an insecticide such as permethrin (Perigen—manufactured by Wellcome as a 10 per cent solution). The edges of the net must be tucked under the mattress during daylight hours, ensuring that no mosquitoes are trapped inside. A needle and thread should be packed as these nets invariably sustain tears.

2. Accommodation with mosquito screening on windows and doors is desirable and it is necessary to be meticulous about closing these screens, especially from late afternoon on. Spraying the rooms with a knock-down insecticide at this time will eliminate any determined invaders who have breached the defences.

3. When out of doors in the evening all family members should wear clothes which cover arms and legs, to reduce the amount of exposed skin. A mosquito repellent such as diethyl toluamide (DEET) is also worth spreading on the skin.

Table 15 Chemoprophylactic regimens against malaria

Regimen	Dose
Cq	Chloroquine 300 mg (2 tablets) weekly*†‡
P	Proguanil 200 mg (2 tablets) daily*‡
CqP	Chloroquine 300 mg (2 tablets) weekly*†‡ Proguanil 200 mg (2 tablets) daily*‡
MaCq	Maloprim (pyrimethamine-dapsone) (1 tablet) weekly*‡§ Chloroquine 300 mg (2 tablets) weekly*†‡
Mf	Mefloquine 250 mg (1 tablet) weekly*‖
O	No chemoprophylaxis¶

* Avoid in severe hepatic and renal impairment.
† Dosages given as mg of chloroquine base. Standard adult tablets of chloroquine contain 150 mg base (equivalent to 200 mg chloroquine sulphate, 250 mg chloroquine phosphate).
‡ Desirable to start one week before departure, essential to continue for four weeks after return.
§ Contraindicated in the first trimester of pregnancy. Give folate supplements if Maloprin is prescribed during second or third trimester. (One Maloprim tablet contains pyrimethamine 12.5 mg and dapsone 100 mg.)
‖ Avoid during pregnancy and lactation; possible risk of interactions with cardioactive agents (β blockers, digoxin, calcium channel blockers) and metoclopramide. Do not prescribe if there is a history of epilepsy or of psychiatric disorder. Not recommended for visits over three weeks abroad (dose change when used for longer visits). Continue tablets weekly after return until the pack of 6 is exhausted. Report side effects to Committee on Safety of Medicines.
¶ Bear in mind remote possibility of malaria if patient presents with fever.

Chemoprophylaxis

The main antimalarials are shown in Tables 15–21, and these may be bought without prescription in some countries. Amodiaquine and Fansidar are no longer recommended for prophylaxis because of serious side-effects. Pyrimethamine on its own (Daraprim) must **not** be used as it seems particularly ineffective in preventing severe falciparum malaria. The malaria reference laboratory published recommended regimes for malaria prophylaxis in 1989 (Reference 13*c* Appendix 6). These are reproduced here; the first 2 tables give the dosages, in adults and children. These are subdivided according to the resistance pattern of the parasite. The next 5 tables include those countries where malaria is prevalent and list the regimes that should be used.

Table 16 Doses of prophylactic antimalarials for children*

Age	Weight (kg)	Fraction of adult dose: Chloroquine/ Proguanil	Maloprim (pyrimethamine-dapsone)	Mefloquine
0–5 weeks		$\frac{1}{8}$	Not recommended	Not recommended
6 weeks–11 months		$\frac{1}{4}$	$\frac{1}{8}$†	Not recommended
1–5 years	10–19	$\frac{1}{2}$	$\frac{1}{4}$	Not recommended (<2 years) $\frac{1}{4}$(2–5 years)
6–11 years	20–39	$\frac{3}{4}$	$\frac{1}{2}$	$\frac{1}{2}$(6–8 years) $\frac{3}{4}$(9–11 years)
>12 years	>40	Adult dose	Adult dose	Adult dose

* When both are available weight is a better guide than age for children over 6 months old.
† Not feasible to prepare unless a paediatric formulation is available.

Table 17 North Africa and Middle East*

Risk extremely low	Risk present, usually low	Risk present
Remember remote chance of malaria if fever presents	Very low risk in major cities	Chloroquine resistance present
Regimen O	*Regimen Cq or P*	*Regimen CqP*
Morocco	Oman	Afghanistan
Algeria	Democratic Yemen	Iran
Tunisia	Egypt (rural, Jun–Oct)	
Libya	Iraq (rural, North, May–Nov)	
	United Arab Emirates (rural)	
	Saudi Arabia (rural)	
Egypt (tourist areas)	Syria (rural, May–Oct)	
	Turkey (rural, Mar–Nov)	
	Yemen (Sep–Feb)	
	Also (outside this area)	
	Mauritius (rural)	

* Transmission confined to rural areas and prophylaxis needed for only part of the year specified in parentheses.

Table 18 Sub Saharan Africa

Very high risk Variable chloroquine resistance	Very high risk Chloroquine resistance	Very high risk Multiple drug resistance
Regimen CqP	*Regimen CqP*	*Regimen CqP* or Mf†*
Benin	Angola	Cameroon
Burkina Faso	Botswana	Kenya
Chad	Burundi	Malawi
Congo	Central African Republic	Tanzania
Equatorial Guinea	Comoros	Uganda
Gabon	Congo	Zaire
Gambia	Djibouti	Zambia
Ghana	Ethiopia	
Guinea	Madagascar	
Guinea-Bissau	Mozambique	
Ivory Coast	Namibia	
Liberia	Rwanda	
Mali	Somalia	
Mauritania	Sudan	
Niger	Swaziland	
Nigeria	Zimbabwe	
Principe	South Africa (only parts of Natal and Transvaal)	
São Tomé		
Senegal		
Sierra-Leone		
Togo		

* CqP needed for frequent, longer term, or pregnant travellers or when regimen Mf is contraindicated.

† Mf is an option only for short term travellers (maximum time abroad three weeks) without contraindications.

Determining the most appropriate regimen for a family is not straightforward. Factors include area of travel, length of stay, and local drug resistance. In such circumstances it is best to consult one of the national advice centres (see Appendix 5). However, it is not recommended to 'shop around' as experts may differ on what is the best regime even in specific circumstances. Medication should be started one week before leaving the UK, be continued throughout the stay in the area, and for **4–6 weeks after return.**

Table 19 Southeast and South Asia

Very low risk Remember chance of malaria if fever	Substantial risk	Risk variable Usually moderate chloroquine resistance present
Regimen O	*Regimen CqP* or Mf†*	*Regimen CqP*
Tourist and cities of:	Thailand (rural)	Bangladesh
Peninsular west Malaysia	West Malaysia	Bhutan
Bali	China (rural, some areas)	India
Thailand	Indonesia (outside Bali)	Nepal
China	Laos	Pakistan
Sarawak	Cambodia	Sri Lanka
Hong Kong	Vietnam	
Philippines	Burma (Myanma)	
Brunei	Philippines (rural)	
Singapore	Sabah	

* CqP needed for frequent, longer term, or pregnant travellers or when regimen Mf is contraindicated.
† Mf is an option only for short term travellers (maximum time abroad three weeks), without contraindications.

Table 20 Oceania

High risk Chloroquine resistance present
Regimen MaCq or Mf†*
Papua New Guinea
Solomon Islands
Vanuatu

* MaCq needed for frequent, longer term, or pregnant travellers or when regimen Mf is contraindicated.
† Mf is an option only for short term travellers (maximum time abroad three weeks), without contraindications.

Table 21 Latin America

Variable risk No chloroquine resistance	Variable or high risk Chloroquine resistance present
Regimen Cq	*Regimen CqP*
Belize	Bolivia (below 2500 m)
Costa Rica (rural)	Brazil (rural, some areas)*
Dominican Republic	Colombia
El Salvador	Ecuador
Guatemala	French Guiana
Haiti	Guyana
Honduras	Panama
Mexico (rural, little visited areas)	Suriname
Nicaragua	Venezuela (rural)
Paraguay (rural, Oct–May)	
Peru (below 1500 m)	
Argentina (a few areas)	

* Amazonas region of Brazil has high risk of chloroquine resistance and regimen Mf is recommended for short term travellers (maximum time abroad three weeks) without contraindications.

The WHO booklet on *Vaccination requirements for international travel* (Further reading, no. 14 Appendix 6) for the current year should be consulted for details of areas within countries (p) and months when malaria transmission (s) occurs.

Hepatitis A

Rates of this infection are highest in travellers returning from Asia and Africa, although anyone consuming impure water or unhygienically prepared food in any country, or living in crowded conditions, is at risk.

Protection

Advise against consumption of high hepatitis-risk shellfish (eg mussels, cockles, oysters) on holiday. Human normal immunoglobulin (HNIG) is highly effective at preventing infection, and dosages for children for protection lasting three or six months are given on p. 165. However, hepatitis in very young children is mild, indeed often asymptomatic, so it is unnecessary to give HNIG to travellers under five. Children (and adults) who repeatedly go to developing countries should have their immunity checked—they may already be immune and can be spared repeated injections. HNIG should be given just before departure and this can cause problems in travellers who present late for their immunoprophylaxis, as it may interfere with immunizations. It is usually advised that HNIG is not given until two weeks after a live virus vaccine, to avoid its reducing the immune response. It has, however, been shown that both individuals who already have some polio immunity (and probably those who don't) and those susceptible to yellow fever mount an adequate response to these vaccines even if HNIG is given simultaneously or up to a week after.

Hepatitis B

See p. 166.

Immunizations less commonly required

Rabies

Three of six cases of imported human rabies between 1977 and 1987 were children, all bitten by dogs in the ISC. Human diploid-cell rabies vaccine (HDCRV) containing inactivated virus is highly effective when administered either pre- or post-exposure and has few side-effects. However, pre-exposure rabies prophylaxis is not routinely recommended for travellers, even those visiting highly endemic zones such as the ISC, Africa, and Latin America. This is because the risk of being bitten by a rabid animal during a short stay is small and when it does occur post-exposure vaccination is highly effective. It should, however, be considered if a family or child is going to a high-risk area where the availability of post-exposure prophylaxis is in doubt. **Specialist consultation is required.** Two injections are needed one month apart and the vaccine is not available on the NHS. It can, however, be given intradermally so that two 1 ml vials (£17 in 1988) will cover a family of four. **Information on this and post-exposure measures are available from Public Health Laboratories, departments of infectious disease, and the CDSC** (Appendix 5, p. 268).

Whether or not pre-exposure vaccine is given, it is essential to educate parents about the risk of rabies which, without post-exposure immunization, is untreatable, causing an agonizing death in virtually 100 per cent of cases. The main risk is from bites, scratches, and licks from dogs, but also cats and any other mammal in the high-risk areas. Though rabies is endemic in other parts of the world, including Europe and North America, it is virtually completely confined to wild animals which normally have the good sense to stay away from children. Children must, however, be discouraged from approaching and handling both wild and domestic animals, especially in Asia and Africa and especially if they are wild cats and dogs. The advice for families is rather complex, as follows.

If a bite, lick, or scratch occurs from an animal that is behaving oddly or looking unwell, the wound must immediately be scrubbed with soap or detergent and running water for at least five minutes, foreign material removed, and then rinsed with plain water. Irrigation with an agent that will kill the virus (eg 0.01% aqueous iodine, povidone iodine, or even gin or whisky—40 per cent alcohol!) further reduces the risk. The child should be taken to a local medical practitioner as soon as possible (**not wait until return to the UK**) and a specific query made about rabies prophylaxis, as well as a tetanus booster if necessary (parents have confused these two). They need to know that rabies prophylaxis is a course of several injections and that the full course is essential. It consists of human rabies immunoglobulin (HRIG) given as soon as possible (20 iu/kg) half irrigating the wound, half intramuscularly. Then a course of human diploid-cell rabies vaccine is started in 1 ml doses, one immediately and then on days 3, 7, 14, 30, and 90. It is given by deep sc injection (away from the site where HRIG was given). In the immunized individual only three injections are needed, one immediately and then on days 7 and 90. **The course may be stopped if the diagnosis is refuted by the animal surviving.**

Meningitis

Meningococcal vaccines are available on prescription against Groups A and C. Their use is dependent on the current epidemiology of meningococcal infection in the world. Thus in 1987 they were recommended for visitors to the Middle East who were going to be living in crowded conditions, because of an epidemic Group A disease in Saudi Arabia associated with pilgrims attending a religious festival. The same argument would apply for visitors to the meningococcal belt in West Africa who will be visiting rural areas.

European tick-borne encephalitis (TBE)

Austria is the most likely country of exposure but the disease occurs from Scandinavia to the Balkans and from Alsace to Western USSR. Most cases of TBE in these countries occur in June and July with a smaller peak in October. It is a serious disease which can cause death or permanent disability. The virus is spread by the common wood tick and the only risk is to persons who trek through or camp near densely forested areas. Some protection is afforded by using stout footwear and an insect repellant. A safe, highly effective unlicensed killed vaccine is available on a named-patient basis from the manufacturers (see below) and further information on its use can be obtained from a national advice centre. Two doses are recommended, at a four- to six-week interval, the second at least two weeks before possible exposure, with a booster at 12 months and three-yearly if there is a continued risk.

Japanese B encephalitis (JBE)

This is prevalent in Southeast Asia and the Far East. A vaccine is available, but is not recommended on a routine basis. A National Advice Centre should be contacted for information. The vaccine is available from Cambridge Selfcare Diagnostic Ltd. (Telephone 091 261 5950).

Travel advice and immunization consultation plan

This will be modified in practice, depending on the child's immunization and medical history, the interval between first consultation and departure, and the proposed itinerary.

1. Six to eight weeks before departure: obtain details of exact itinerary, lifestyle, and past immunization history. From this, plan immunization required. If appropriate, start with:

BCG (after tuberculin test);
typhoid;

tetanus booster;
arrange/advise yellow fever for 4 weeks' time at nearest centre;
appointment for OPV booster at **same time**.

2. Two to four weeks before departure:

Confirm yellow fever given;
if indicated, administer: measles, OPV, second typhoid, second cholera;
give general advice about hygiene, food, water, rabies.

3. A week before departure: if indicated, immunoglobulin (HNIG).

The child travelling from abroad

The two main groups are families returning from a short stay in Europe or the Mediterranean, and travellers from the Indian subcontinent or Africa (West or East), either after a long stay or as new immigrants.

The child with an infection most commonly presents with fever and/or gastrointestinal symptoms. Some points to consider for any child (or adult) recently returned are:

1. Any fever in such a person or a contact requires urgent investigation. Many travel-acquired infections have implications for contacts and are notifiable. Also, not all imported infections occur clinically in the traveller. The first case may be in a UK contact who has never been abroad. Examples of this have occurred for meningococcal meningitis type A, typhoid, polio, diphtheria, hepatitis A, and non-enteric salmonellosis.

2. Not all imported infections are necessarily exotic: the commonest are gastroenteritis due to *Salmonella*, *Campylobacter*, *Shigella*, and *E. coli*.

3. There should be a higher diagnostic suspicion for diseases which used to be prevalent in UK children, such as diphtheria, polio, and tuberculosis, especially in children of im-

migrants entering the country for the first time or who may have been away on extended visits and whose immunizations are likely to be less than required.

4. Most new immigrants will be underimmunized (parents as well as children).

Diagnosis and public-health management

The individual coming from abroad could have almost any infectious disease and space precludes detailed reference to all possibilities. The BMA publish a useful guide (see Further reading, no. 12 Appendix 6). Benenson's guide (Further reading, no. 2) is also highly recommended, though it only comes into its own once the diagnosis has been made.

Some pointers for action are:

1. Take a country-by-country history with dates (of family contacts if the child has not recently been abroad) and consult a specialist.

2. Malaria must be considered in a child who has been in an endemic zone, however long ago. It may be falciparum, which can kill if not treated early.

3. If malaria can be excluded in a **fever** with non-specific symptoms and/or rash, consider typhoid, hepatitis A, meningococcal infection, or tuberculosis. There is always concern about Lassa fever in returnees from West Africa. However, none of the 10 importations 1971–87 have been in children, although it does occur at young ages in endemic zones. The common bacterial causes of **gastroenteritis** are listed on p. 60. A profuse watery diarrhoea may be due to cholera. Prolonged diarrhoea and non-specific abdominal symptoms may be caused by *Giardia lamblia*. It is also important to look for some of the intestinal worms, both exotic and commonplace. This can be done by a stool specimen, requesting microscopy and detailing the country of origin.

4. If there is **fever and sore throat**, consider diphtheria, and look for weeping skin lesions among close contacts, which may be cutaneous diphtheria. If **fever is combined with neurological symptoms**, typhoid, malaria and meningitis may present this way; also consider rabies. Poliomyelitis may be the cause of aseptic meningitis or a febrile illness with paralysis in a recent

returnee. With **fever and jaundice** the commonest causes are viral hepatitis and falciparum malaria. A rare possibility in a very sick patient is yellow fever.

Post-holiday rabies concerns

Increasing public awareness of rabies and foreign travel has led to increasing demand for advice about possible exposure. The following history should be taken:

1. Personal. Name, age, sex, weight, address of the child, and family telephone number.

2. The exposure. Type (bite/lick/scratch, etc.). Where on the body? Was the skin broken? (Examine the site.) When did it occur and what was the exact geographic location? Details of local advice or management of the wound, including name, site, and number of vaccinations given.

3. The animal. Species, wild or domestic? Name, telephone number, and address of owners known? Was the animal provoked (eg child teasing it), and was it behaving oddly? Did it look ill? What happened to it subsequently? **If the animal was known to be alive 14 days after the bite, rabies can be excluded.**

4. Were local public health authorities informed? Was the animal's brain being examined? If so, appropriate names, addresses, and telephone numbers.

There will be some circumstances, e.g. dog-bite in India, where the high risk will be clear and post-exposure prophylaxis with human rabies immunoglobulin (HRIG) (half around wound, half intra-muscular) and HDCRV (into upper arm, not buttock) must be started immediately. A delay of weeks or even months after an exposure is **not** a contraindication to prophylaxis. Domestic animals can often be traced through local British Embassies via DHSS International Division (consult DH direct (071–470 1255) or the CDSC (081–200 6868) may advise.

A short list of the actions to be taken for these important diseases is shown in Table 22.

Table 22 Major health actions needed for principal serious imported diseases in the UK

Infection	Notifiable	Public-health measures in UK	Reference
Typhoid and paratyphoid	Yes*	Case should be isolated Screen household contacts. Exclusion from nursery/infant school until 3 negative stool and urine specimens at weekly intervals beginning after clinical recovery; hygiene education.	PHLS salmonella subcommittee: Notes on the control of human sources of gastrointestinal infections, infestations, and bacterial intoxications in the UK available from PHLS CDSC
Cholera	Yes* but only if *V. cholerae* 01 isolated (often non-cholera vibrios can cause watery diarrhoea)	Case isolated. Clinical surveillance of household contacts for 5 days after last exposure to case or source; hygiene education. NB: no risk of epidemic cholera in UK.	
Malaria	Yes	None	—
Yellow fever	Yes	None	—
Rabies	Yes*	Patient admitted to high-security unit. Close contacts offered post-exposure vaccination	DH memorandum on Rabies, 1977. London: HMSO
Viral haemorrhagic fever (Lassa, Marburg, Ebola)	Yes*	Patient admitted to high-security unit. Clinical surveillance of close contacts	DH memorandum on the control of viral haemorrhagic fevers, 1986. London: HMSO

* For all suspected or confirmed cases also inform CDSC by telephone: 081–200 6868 (24 hours and weekends), ask for duty doctor. For Scotland: CD(S)H, Tel.: 041–946 7120.

Appendices

Appendix 1

Notifiable diseases (as at 1 August 1990)

	England and Wales	Northern Ireland	Scotland
Acute encephalitis	+	+	0
Acute poliomyelitis	+	+	+
Anthrax	+	+	+
Chickenpox	0	0	+
Cholera	+	+	+
Diphtheria	+	+	+
Dysentery (amoebic or bacillary)	+	+	+
Erysipelas	0	0	+
Food poisoning (all sources)	+	+	+
Legionella	0	0	+
Leprosy	+	0	+
Leptospirosis	+	0	Leptospiral jaundice
Malaria	+	0	+
Measles	+	+	+
Membranous croup	0	0	+
Meningitis	+	+	0
Meningococcal septicaemia (without meningitis)	+	+	+
Mumps	+	+	+

Ophthalmia neonatorum, includes *Neisseria gonorrhoeae* and *Chlamydia trachomatis* infection	+	0	+
Paratyphoid fever	+	+	+
Plague	+	+	+
Puerperal fever	0	0	+
Rabies	+	+	+
Relapsing fever	+	+	+
Rubella	+	+	+
Scarlet fever	+	+	+
Smallpox	+	+	+
Tetanus	+	0	0
Tuberculosis	+	+	+
Typhoid fever	+	+	+
Typhus	+	+	+
Viral haemorrhagic fever	+	+	+
Viral hepatitis	+	+	+
Whooping cough	+	+	+
Yellow fever	+	+	+
Notify	Medical Officer of Environmental Health of the local authority (or officer performing his function)	Chief Administrative Medical Officer of the appropriate Health and Social Services Board	Chief Administrative Medical Officer of the appropriate Health Board

Report AIDS cases on a special AIDS Clinical Report Form in strict medical confidence to the Director, PHLS CDSC, 61 Colinsdale Avenue, London NW9 5EQ.

Appendix 2

Anti-microbials

Bold typescript indicates individual dosage on body weight or surface area basis, the higher dose for severe infections (e.g. meningitis)

Drug	Route	Times Daily	Usual individual dosage				Comments
			Birth*	1 year	7 years	14 years	
Acyclovir	iv o	3 5	**15 mg/kg** —		**250–500 mg/m²** 200–400 mg		Zovirax: used for severe neo-natal HSV infection, herpes encephalitis, eczema herpeticum, and varicella in immunocompromised children. Higher doses in herpes encephalitis and immunocompromised.
Amikacin	iv	2			**7.5 mg/kg**		Amikin: aminoglycoside sometimes used for severe Gram-negative infections, i.e. cystic fibrosis. Atypical TB. Check renal function prior to use. Weekly drug levels. Check hearing regularly even when drug levels normal.
Amoxycillin	o iv	3	31 mg	62.5 mg	125 mg	250 mg	Amoxil: treatment of otitis media, pneumonia, etc; standard course 5 days. **100 mg/kg (for meningitis).** For im use mix with 1% lignocaine instead of water.

Amoxycillin and clavulanic acid	o iv	3	31 mg	62.5 mg	125 mg	250 mg	Augmentin: clavulanic acid is beta-lactamase inhibitor; broadens spectrum of amoxycillin to include most *Staphylococcus aureus* and other penicillinase-producing strains.
Amphotericin	iv (infuse over 6 hours)	1		250 micrograms/kg			Fungizone: fungal, esp. candidal septicaemia, usually in neonate or immunocompromised child. Increase dose gradually over several days to 1 mg/kg. Several weeks' therapy may be required. Watch renal tubular function. Check levels.
Ampicillin	o iv	4	62.5 mg tds	125 mg **50–100 mg/kg**	250 mg	500 mg	Penbritin: otitis media, pneumonia, and meningitis.
Azlocillin	iv	3	**150 mg/kg to maximum of 3 g**				Securopen: treatment of pseudomonas septicaemia in the immunocompromised child and cystic fibrosis. Contraindicated in penicillin allergy.
Aztreonam	iv	3–4	—	**30–50 mg/kg** to maximum of 8 g			Azactam: a monocyclic beta lactam. Active against Gram negative bacteria including *Pseudomonas aeruginosa*, *Haemophilus influenzae*. Low risk of hypersensitivity in children with penicillin allergy.

* Special care should be taken in prescribing antibiotics in the neonatal period, particularly for preterm infants and specialist texts should be consulted in this situation, as the dosages given may not be appropriate in all circumstances.

Key: bd = twice daily; tds = three times daily; qds = four times daily.

Drug	Route	Times Daily	Usual individual dosage				Comments
			Birth*	1 year	7 years	14 years	
Benzylpenicillin		See penicillin G					
Cefotaxime	iv	3–4	**50 mg/kg** < 1 wk bd > 1 wk tds	**25–50 mg/kg**			Claforan: treatment of septicaemia, meningitis, and life-threatening infections. Reduce dose in renal failure. Max. doses in meningitis.
Ceftazidime	iv	3	**12.5–30 mg/kg (bd)**	**25–50 mg/kg**			Fortum: broad spectrum. Particularly effective in *Pseudomonas aeruginosa* infections. Use high dose in children with cystic fibrosis, meningitis, and the immunocompromized.
Cefuroxime	iv	3	**20–40 mg/kg (< 1 wk bd)**	**25–50 mg/kg**			Zinacef: *H. influenzae* infections and neonatal sepsis. Reduce dose in renal impairment.
Cephradine	o iv im	4	—	**25–50 mg/kg**			Velosef: treatment of infections, i.e. orthopaedic and urine infections if resistant organisms. Reduce dose in renal impairment.

Chloramphenicol	o iv	4	(see neonatal vade-mecum)	**25 mg/kg for 48 hours then 12.5 mg/kg**			Chloromycetin: only used for treatment of meningitis, epiglottitis, and some cases of typhoid. Monitor levels in neonates and in children having concurrent phenobarbitone. High dose ampicillin/penicillin G can be substituted if organism sensitive to these drugs. Well absorbed orally.
Chloroquine	o	Initially **10 mg/kg** to a maximum of **600 mg**; 6 hours later **5 mg/kg**; then **5 mg/kg** per day, daily dose for 2 days					Avloclor: initial treatment of simple malaria when chloroquine resistance is not a problem.
Ciprofloxacin	o iv	2	—	**3.75–7.5 mg/kg**			Ciproxin: Pseudomonas infection in cystic fibrosis. iv preparation not recommended
Clindamycin	o iv	4 3–4	— —	**3–6 mg/kg** **5–10 mg/kg**			Dalacin: arthropathy in animal studies. Staphylococcal bone and joint infection. Watch for pseudomembranous colitis
Clotrimazole	o	3	Use topically				Fungal infection—*Tinea pedis* (athlete's foot)
Co-trimoxazole	o	2	—	240 mg/kg	480 mg/kg	960 mg/kg	Bactrim/Septrin: urinary tract infections, chest infections, typhoid, invasive salmonellosis. Drug is mixture of 5 parts sulphamethoxazole and 1 part trimethoprim (dose = sum of each in mg)
			48 mg/kg as urinary-tract infection prophylaxis at night.				
	iv	4	**30 mg/kg for *Pneumocystis carinii* pneumonia**				

Drug	Route	Times Daily	Usual individual dosage				Comments
			Birth*	1 year	7 years	14 years	
Diethylcarbamazine	o	2		**0.5–3 mg/kg**			Banocide: filariasis.
Erythromycin	o	4	< 1 wk **10 mg/kg**	125 mg	250 mg	500 mg	Erythroped: use when definite history of penicillin allergy.
as lactobionate	iv	4	—		**12.5–25 mg/kg**		Treatment of *Chlamydia trachomatis*, *C. psittaci*, *Legionella*, and *Mycoplasma pneumoniae* infection.
Ethambutol	o	1	—	—	**25 mg/kg**		Myambutol: treatment of tuberculosis. Used in conjunction with isoniazid and/or rifampicin. Avoid in renal impairment. Visual problems can result and it should not be given to children < 6 yr. Test colour vision before and during treatment. Reduce dose after 60 days to 15 mg/kg/day if still required
Flucloxacillin **or Cloxacillin**	o iv	4	62.5 mg	125 mg **25–50 mg/kg**	250 mg	500 mg	Floxapen: staphylococcal infections—septicaemia and osteomyelitis. May be combined with another antibiotic. Drain any abscess surgically.

Fluconazole	o iv	1 1		**3–6 mg/kg**			Diflucan: little experience of use in children. For systemic candidiasis and cryptococcal infection. Reduce dose in renal impairment.
Flucytosine	o iv	4 4		**25–50 mg/kg**			Alcoban: for systemic candidiasis and cryptococcosis.
Fusidic acid	o	3	—	250 mg (as fusidic acid)	500 mg	750 mg	Fucidin: osteomyelitis and suppurative arthritis. Life threatening *Staphylococcus aureus* infection.
	iv	3			6 mg/kg (as sodium fusidate)		May be combined with flucloxacillin or erythromycin.
Gentamicin	iv	3	**2.5 mg/kg** bd < 1 wk; tds > 1 wk		**2.5 mg/kg**		Genticin: Gram-negative infections, neonatal sepsis, cystic fibrosis. Always monitor trough and peak levels. Aim for peak less than 10 mg/l and trough under 2 mg/l. Children with cystic fibrosis need higher doses.
Griseofulvin	o	2	—		**5 mg/kg**		For ringworm of scalp (6 weeks); nails (6 months). May cause photosensitivity.
Imipenem with cilastin	iv	4		**15 mg/kg** (Max. 2 g/day)			Primaxin: a thienamycin beta lactam antibiotic. For aerobic and anaerobic Gram positive and negative bacteria.

Drug	Route	Times Daily	Usual individual dosage				Comments
			Birth*	1 year	7 years	14 years	
Isoniazid	o im iv	1	**3–10 mg/kg**	**10 mg/kg**	**200 mg**	**300 mg**	Treatment of tuberculosis. Combined with other drugs unless for prophylaxis. Give pyridoxine to prevent peripheral neuritis. **For TB meningitis** use 10–20 mg/kg.
Mebendazole	o	1	—	—	100 mg if 2 yrs and older		Vermox: for hookworm infections. Contraindicated in children under 2 years of age.
Metronidazole	o	1		500 mg	1 g	2 g	Flagyl: giardiasis. 3 days' treatment.
		3		200 mg	400 mg	800 mg	Amoebiasis. Treat for 5 days.
	pr	3	—	250 mg	500 mg	1 g	Anaerobic infection.
	iv (20 min)	3		**7.5 mg/kg**			
Miconazole	o iv (30 min)	4 3	62.5 mg	62.5 mg **12–15 mg/kg**	125 mg	125–250 mg	Daktarin: fungal infections esp. *Candida*. Oral preparation for oral thrush. Discuss with microbiologist before using for systemic candidiasis.
Netilmicin	iv im	3	**2.5 mg/kg bd < 1 wk; tds > 1 wk**		**2.5 mg/kg**		Netillin: Gram-negative infections. Neonatal sepsis, cystic fibrosis. Always monitor levels. Children with cystic fibrosis need higher dosage.

Nitrofurantoin	o	4	Avoid in neonatal period		**0.75 mg/kg**		For urinary-tract infections with multiple organism resistance. May cause nausea and vomiting.
Nystatin	o topical	3 or 4		100 000 U			Given for oral thrush or infantile eczema infected with *Candida*.
Penicillin G (benzylpenicillin)	im iv	4 **4–6**	50 mg/kg	150 mg **25–50 mg/kg** **Higher dose** **4-hourly in meningitis** **and endocarditis**	300 mg	600 mg	Crystapen: 1 megaunit = 600 mg. Tonsillitis, lobar pneumonia, erysipelas, endocarditis, meningococcal, and pneumococcal meningitis.
Penicillin G—Domiciliary use emergency treatment of meningococcal infection				600 mg	1200 mg	1200 mg	
Penicillin G as procaine penicillin	im	1		60 mg/kg to maximum of 2.4 g			For treatment of gonococcal infection in childhood. Therapeutic level maintained better with Probenecid given 30 minutes before injection (1 gm oral).
Penicillin V (phenoxymethyl-penicillin)	o	4	62.5 mg	125 mg	250 mg	500 mg	Tonsillitis Tonsillitis and minor infections, prophylaxis of rheumatic fever and septicaemia after splenectomy. Pneumonia after initial iv/im penicillin. Prophylactic usage can be given once or twice daily in doses shown.

Drug	Route	Times Daily	Usual individual dosage				Comments
			Birth*	1 year	7 years	14 years	
Piperacillin	iv	4	50–100 mg (bd) or tds		**50–75 mg/kg**		Pipril: for treatment of *Pseudomonas aeruginosa* infection in children with cystic fibrosis. Combine with aminoglycoside.
Piperazine	o	Single doses given 14 days apart (×2)	< 1 y $\frac{1}{3}$ sachet	$\frac{2}{3}$ sachet	1 sachet		Pripsen: for treatment of threadworms.
Pivampicillin	o	3		175 mg	175 mg	250 mg	Pondocillin: 175 mg in 5 ml. Similar antibacterial spectrum as ampicillin, with better absorption.
Pyrazinamide	o	3	—		**7–12 mg/kg**		Zinamide: used in tuberculous meningitis. Not licensed for use in children in UK. Watch liver function.
Pyrimethamine	o (give folinic acid supplement)	1	**1 mg/kg**				In combination with sulphadiazine for congenital toxoplasmosis in 3-week course alternating with spiramycin.

Quinine	o iv (over 4 h)	3 3	60 mg	125 mg **10 mg/kg**	300 mg	600 mg	Doses given as base. Quinine base, 100 mg = quinine bisulphate; 169 mg = quinine dihydrochloride/hydrochloride or quinine sulphate 122 mg. Treatment of malaria, esp. if chloroquine resistance, or cerebral malaria. With resistant strains an iv loading dose of 20 mg/kg is required, switch to oral therapy as soon as possible. Always seek specialist advice. Treatment usually given for 10–14 days. iv therapy only given > 3 months, oral from birth.
Rifampicin	o iv	1	**10 mg/kg**	**20 mg/kg** (maximum dosage 600 mg)	600 mg	600 mg	Rifadin: treatment of tuberculosis.
Rifampicin	o	2 (for 2 days)	**5 mg/kg**	**10 mg/kg**	**10 mg/kg**	600 mg	Prophylaxis of *Neisseria meningitidis* infection.
as prophylaxis	o	1 (for 4 days)	**10 mg/kg**	**20 mg/kg to maximum of 600 mg**			Prophylaxis of *Haemophilus influenzae* infection, etc. Drug interaction with oral contraceptive and chloramphenicol. Warn about orange secretions.
Spiramycin	o	2		1–2 g			For treatment of cryptosporidiosis in the immunosuppressed.
	o	2	**50 mg/kg**				Congenital toxoplasmosis. Alone, or alternating with pyrimethamine and sulphadiazine in 3-weekly cycles.

Drug	Route	Times Daily	Usual individual dosage				Comments
			Birth*	1 year	7 years	14 years	
Streptomycin	im	1	—	**30–40 mg/kg**	**30–40 mg/kg**	1 g	Treatment of tuberculous meningitis for first few weeks (not more than 12). Other antituberculous drugs also always given simultaneously.
Sulphadiazine	o	2	**50 mg/kg**				Congenital toxoplasmosis in combination with pyrimethamine alternated with spiramycin in 3-weekly cycles.
Thiabendazole	o	2			**25 mg/kg**		Mintezol: treatment of refractory hookworm, threadworm, whipworm, roundworm, visceral larva migrans, *Strongyloides*. Treatment given for 2–7 days—see literature.
Tobramycin	iv	3	—		**2.5 mg/kg**		Monitor levels; ototoxic. Treatment of gram-negative infection in the immunosuppressed.
Trimethoprim	o	2	avoid in neonatal period	50 mg	100 mg	200 mg	For urinary-tract infections.
	iv	2			**3–4.5 mg/kg**		Single evening dose as prophylaxis **1–2 mg/kg**.

Vancomycin	iv	2–4	15 mg/kg dose once. Then 10 mg/kg 12-hourly under 1 week, or 15 mg/kg dose once then 10 mg/kg 8-hourly 1–4 weeks	44 mg/kg/day	Use in multiple resistant staphylococcal infections. Very expensive. Ototoxic nephrotoxic. Check levels.

* Special care should be taken in prescribing antibiotics in the neonatal period, particularly for preterm infants and specialist texts should be consulted in this situation, as the dosages given may not be appropriate in all circumstances.

Key: bd = twice daily; tds = three times daily; qds = four times daily.

Appendix 3

Rapid guide to exclusion periods

(See also main text. Note: includes some illnesses not described in text.)

Disease	Incubation period (time from meeting organisms to first symptoms)	
	Common range	Extreme range
Amoebic dysentery*	Variable, commonly 2–4 weeks	
Campylobacter gastroenteritis	3–5 days	1–10 days
Chickenpox	13–17 days	13–21 days
Cholera*	2–3 days	few hours to 5 days
Diphtheria*	2–5 days	2–7 days
E. coli	1–6 days	
Fifth disease	5–22 days	
Gastroenteritis: *Campylobacter*/rotavirus/*Shigella*/typhoid—see individual notes		
Giardiasis	Variable 5–25 days	—
Glandular fever	4–6 weeks	—

Infectious period (when child may pass on disease)	Type of spread and infectivity (how easily child can pass on the disease)	Exclusion period (from school nursery etc.)
May be prolonged	Food/water, faecal hand–mouth Inf: Moderate	(MOEH) Until 3 stool specimens negative for cysts
Infectious throughout illness—until antibiotic given	Food/water faecal hand–mouth Inf: Moderate	Until asymptomatic
1–2 days before rash appears to 6 days after rash first appears	Nearby persons—droplet or contact Inf: High n.b. Danger to immuno-suppressed	Until 6 days from appearance of rash and vesicles have crusted
Variable—until stools are negative	Contaminated food or water Inf: High	(MOEH)
Variable; usually 2–4 weeks from first signs There are carriers	Nearby persons—contact Inf: Moderate	(MOEH)
Variable; may be prolonged beyond diarrhoea	Faecal hand–mouth Inf: Moderate	(MOEH)
Unknown	Unclear	None
During symptoms There are carriers	Faecal hand–mouth Inf: Low	None
Prolonged beyond illness There are carriers	Very close contact Inf: Low	Nil for schoolchildren

Disease	Incubation period (time from meeting organisms to first symptoms)	
	Common range	Extreme range
Hand, foot, and mouth disease (Coxsackie virus)	3–5 days	—
Headlice (see nits)		—
Hepatitis A* (infectious hepatitis)	28–30 days	15–50 days
Hepatitis B* (serum H)	60–90 days	45–160 days
Herpes simplex (cold sores)	2–12 days	—
Impetigo—streptococcal/	1–3 days	—
staphylococcal	4–10 days	—
Influenza	2–3 days	—
Malaria*	12–30 days	8–10 months from one rare type
Measles*	8–13 days to fever 10–15 days to rash	—
Meningococcal disease*	3–4 days	2–10 days
Molluscum contagiosum	2–7 weeks	—

Infectious period (when child may pass on disease)	Type of spread and infectivity (how easily child can pass on the disease)	Exclusion period (from school nursery etc.)
Acute phase of illness	Nearby persons—contact, faecal hand–mouth and droplet Inf: Low	During acute phase of illness
—	High	None
14 days before jaundice to 7 days after	Contact by hand, faecal, oral, and contaminated food or water Inf: Moderate	7 days from jaundice starting
Infectious before and after illness There are carriers	Very close contact or contaminated blood Inf: Very low	Nil once well
Variable	Close contact Inf: Moderate	Nil
While lesions are draining	By contact Inf: High	Until lesions have healed
The 3 days before onset of symptoms	Nearby persons by droplet Inf: High	Nil once well
—	Not infectious in UK	Nil
From first symptoms until 4 days after rash appears	Nearby persons—droplet Inf: Very high	Until 4 days after appearance of rash Danger to immunocompromised
Low risk after 2 days of rash	Low	Nil
There are carriers	Nearby persons—droplet	recommend rifampicin prophylaxis Seek advice (MOEH)
As long as lesions persist	Very close contact Inf: Very low	Nil

Disease	Incubation period (time from meeting organisms to first symptoms)	
	Common range	Extreme range
Mumps*	18 days	14–21 days
Nits/head lice (*Pediculosis capitis*)	7 days	—
Polio*	7–14 days	3–35 days
Ringworm (scalp)	10–14 days	—
Ringworm (body)	4–10 days	—
Ringworm (feet) (athletes' foot)	Unknown	—
Rotavirus	48 h approx.	—
Rubella**	16–18 days	14–23 days
Scabies	days to weeks	—
Shigella* (bacillary dysentery)	1–3 days	1–7 days
Tetanus*	4–10 days	4–21 days
Tuberculosis*	4–12 weeks	—
Typhoid*	1–3 weeks	—
Warts and verrucae	4 months	1–12 months

Infectious period (when child may pass on disease)	Type of spread and infectivity (how easily child can pass on the disease)	Exclusion period (from school nursery etc.)
6 days before swelling to 9 days after	Nearby contact—droplet	None
Max. 2 days before swelling	Inf: High	
As long as lice remain alive or hair is untreated	Very close contact Inf: Low	Only if parents refuse to treat child
Via faeces for 3–6 weeks	Nearby—faeces, hand, mouth Inf: High	Seek advice (MOEH)
As long as lesions are present	All by direct contact Inf: Low	None
When symptomatic	Faecal hand–mouth Inf: Moderate	Until 72 hours of diarrhoea ceases
7 days before rash until 4 days after	Nearby—droplet or contact Inf: High	Until 4 days after rash appears
Until mites and eggs destroyed by two treatments	Very close contact Inf: Low	Until after treatment has started
Usually while symptomatic and in the carrier state	Faecal, hand–mouth Inf: High	Until 3 stool specimens negative (MOEH)
No person-to-person spread	From soil Inf: Nil	Nil
Variable	By close contact Inf: Low	(MOEH and chest physician)
Until stool clear	Faecal hand–mouth Inf: Moderate	Until 3 stools negative
Unknown, possibly as long as lesion lasts	Very close contact Inf: V. low	Nil

Disease	Incubation period (time from meeting organisms to first symptoms)	
	Common range	Extreme range
Whooping cough*	7–10 days	7–21 days

* Notifiable disease.
** see congenital rubella (p. 106) *re* notification.
MOEH Consultation with Medical Officer of Environmental Health (or alternative
Note: Information on gastrointestinal infection derived from Communicable Disease

Infectious period (when child may pass on disease)	Type of spread and infectivity (how easily child can pass on the disease)	Exclusion period (from school nursery etc.)
Up to 3 weeks after paroxysmal coughing starts or until 7 days after antibiotic commences	Droplet Inf: High	5 days from starting antibiotic treatment

officer) advised.
Report, Supplement 1, 1990 (see Further reading, Appendix 6).

Appendix 4

NATIONAL IMMUNIZATION SCHEDULE (subject to usual contraindications)

Pre-school

Birth	BCG for babies in Asian and other immigrant families with high TB rates and those in contact with active respiratory tuberculosis
2 months	Polio + diphtheria/tetanus/pertussis (DTP)
3 months	Polio + DTP
4 months	Polio + DTP
12–18 months (preferably at 15 months)	Combined measles, mumps, and rubella (MMR) or measles

Pre-school

4–5 years	MMR, if not previously given, + polio + diphtheria/tetanus booster

Secondary school

10–14 years	Heaf or Mantoux and, if negative, BCG
10–14 years	Rubella (girls only)

School leaving

15–19 years	Polio + Tetanus

Schedules for unimmunized children

(Primary schedule for an unimmunized child (subject to the usual contraindications)

Under 3	First injection MMR (or measles) + diphtheria/tetanus/pertussis (DTP) + polio After 1 month DTP + polio After another 1 month DTP + polio Booster after 3 years

Age 3–6th birthday	First injection MMR or (measles) + DTP + polio After 1 month DTP + polio After another month DTP + polio Booster after 3 years
Age 6–10th birthday	First injection MMR (or measles) + DTP* or Dip/Tet* + polio After 1 month DTP* or Dip/Tet* + polio After another month DTP* or Dip/Tet* + polio Booster after 3 years
Over 10	Consider Heaf/Mantoux (Asian child) First injection MMR (or measles) + low-dose diphtheria** (see p. 164) + tetanus + polio After 1 month low-dose diphtheria + tetanus + polio After another month low-dose diphtheria + tetanus + polio

Girls over 14 also need a rubella injection if they have not had one.

* Where young siblings are at risk of catching whooping cough older children should be offered DTP not diphtheria/tetanus.

Note: Three years should elapse between giving the primary course and the pre-school booster of diphtheria/tetanus and polio.

** This requires three injections at the first visit, which is asking a lot of the child's and the parents' stamina. It may be best to leave out diphtheria on the first occasion and give a third dose one month after stage 3.

Schedules for catching up with whooping cough

Schedule for catching up with whooping cough, e.g. where parents have decided they want their child to have the injection having missed out beforehand.

For all ages	First injection pertussis (monovalent) After 1 month pertussis After another 1 month pertussis

Appendix 5

SOURCES OF SPECIALIST ADVICE

Public Health Laboratories

England and Wales

Central PHLS, Communicable Disease Surveillance Centre, Tel.: 081 200 6868.

PHLS Virus Reference Laboratory, Tel.: 081 200 4400

PHL Ashford	0223 635731
PHL Bath	0225 823266
PHL Birmingham	021 772 3009
PHL Brighton	0273 696955
PHL Bristol	0272 291326
PHL Cambridge	0223 242111
PHL Cardiff	0222 755944
PHL Dorchester	0305 251150
PHL Epsom	03727 26633
PHL Exeter	0392 402972
PHL Gloucester	0452 305334
PHL Guildford	0483 66091
PHL Leeds	0532 645011
PHL Liverpool	051 525 2323
PHL Luton	0582 490890
PHL Newcastle	091 273 8811
PHL Norwich	0603 611816
PHL Nottingham	0602 709163
PHL Oxford	0865 60631
PHL Poole	0202 675771
PHL Portsmouth	0705 822331
PHL Sheffield	0742 437749
PHL Swansea	0792 205666
PHL Taunton	0823 335577
PHL Watford	0923 244366

Scotland

Doctors should contact local laboratories, Health Board Communicable Disease Centre Departments, or the Communicable Disease (Scotland) Unit, Tel.: 041 946 7120.

Information centres for travel

These prefer telephone consultations from the patient's doctor.

England

Public Health Laboratory Service,
Communicable Disease Surveillance Centre,
61 Colindale Avenue,
London NW9 5EQ.
Tel.: 081 200 6868 (ask for duty doctor)

Wales

Welsh Office,
Cathays Park,
Cardiff CF1 3NQ.
Tel.: 0222 82511, Ext. 3336

Scotland

Scottish Home and Health Dept,
St Andrew's House,
Edinburgh EH1 3DE.
Tel.: 031 556 8501, Ext. 2438

The Communicable Disease (Scotland) Unit,
Ruchill Hospital,
Bilsland Drive,
Glasgow G20 9NB.
Tel.: 041 946 7120

Northern Ireland

DHSS, Dundonald House,
Upper Newtownards Road,
Belfast BT4 3SF.
Tel.: 0232 63939, Ext. 2593

For post-exposure rabies prophylaxis course and advice, Tel.: 0232 65011, Ext. 758.

Other centres

Malaria Reference Laboratory,
London School of Hygiene and Tropical Medicine,
Keppel Street,
London WC1E 7HT.
Tel.: 071 636 7921

Medical Advisory Reference for Travellers Abroad (MASTA),
Bureau of Hygiene and Tropical Diseases,
Keppel Street,
London WC1E 7HT.
Tel.: 071 631 4408

British Airways Medical Centre,
75 Regent Street,
London W1.
Tel.: 071 434 4720

Provides advice to public and profession immunization service (all vaccines available).

Appendix 6

FURTHER READING

Infectious diseases

1. Krugman, S., Katz, S. L., Gershon, A. A. and Wilfert, C. M. (1985). *Infectious diseases of children.* CV Mosby, St. Louis.
   American, highly detailed tome.
2. Benenson, A. S. (1985). *Control of communicable diseases in man,* (14th edn). American Public Health Association, Washington.
   An excellent practical handbook.
3. Farrar, W. E. and Lambert, H. P. (1984). *Infectious diseases.* Gower, London.
   A short pictorial guide including most of the common rashes.
4. Emond, R. T. D. and Rowland, H. A. K. (1987). *Colour atlas of infectious diseases,* (2nd edn). Wolfe Medical Atlas.
   A more complete pictorial guide.
5. Public Health Laboratory Service Communicable Disease Surveillance Centre (1990). *Notes on the control of human sources of gastrointestinal infections, infestations and bacterial intoxications in the United Kingdom.* Communicable Disease Report, Supplement 1.
6. *Report of the Committee on Infectious Diseases, American Academy of Pediatrics* ('The Red Book'), (20th edn) (1986).
   To acquire this very complete guide to infectious diseases and immunizations it may be necessary to write to the American Academy, 141 Northwest Point Boulevard, PO Box 927, Elk Grove Village, Illinois 60007, USA.

Immunizations

7. *Immunization against infectious disease* (1990). DHSS.
8. *British national formulary.* BMA/Pharmaceutical Society.
   Regularly updated and collects all vaccines into a handy section. Issued free to all doctors.
9. *Data sheet compendium.* Association of the British Pharmaceutical Industry, London.
   Updated annually, collates all the current data-sheets but not in a single section for immunizations. Issued free to all doctors. Data-sheets tend to be over-cautious with regard to vaccine recommendations.

Immunoglobulins

10. Indications and dosage for normal and special immunoglobulins. Blood Products Laboratory, Elstree, Middlesex. Unpublished. Available from PHLS.

Travel abroad

11. Dawood, R. (ed.) (1986). *Travellers' health.* Oxford University Press. A guide for the layman but also useful for doctors.
12. Walker, E. and Williams, G. (1985). *ABC of health travel,* (2nd edn). British Medical Association, London.
13. (a) *The travellers guide to health.* Leaflet T1
    Available: travel agents. Middx HA7 1AY. Updated annually, gives the current vaccination requirements of all countries.
    (b) *Travel information for medical practitioners* (El 89. p. 33).
    Both publications available from Health Publications Unit, No. 2 Site, Heywood Stores, Manchester Road, Heywood, Lancs. OL10 2PZ (0800 555777)
    (c) from Travel abroad section Prophylaxis against malaria for travellers from the United Kingdom. Bradley, DJ, Phillips Howard, PA. British Medical Journal. 1989; 299: 1087–9.
14. *Vaccination requirements and health advice for international travel,* (1988). WHO, Geneva.
    Available from HMSO.

Official statistics England and Wales

15. Office of Population Censuses and Surveys: Annual Monitors

Series no.	Subject
DH2	Mortality by cause
DH3	Childhood and maternity mortality statistics
MB2	Infectious diseases

Available in good medical libraries and for purchase from HMSO.
OPCS weekly monitors

16. *Communicable Disease Reports.* Published weekly by the Communicative Disease Surveillance Centre.

Human Immunodeficiency Virus (HIV)

17. Batty, D. (ed.) (1987). *The implications of AIDS for children in care.* BAAF.

Available from the British Agency for Adoption and Fostering, 11 Southwark Street, London SE1 1RQ.

18. The Royal College of Obstetricians and Gynaecologists. *Report of the RCOG sub-committee on problems associated wth AIDS in relation to obstetrics and gynaecology.*
Available from the RCOG, 27 Sussex Place, London NW1 4RG. A guide to practical management problems for obstetricians, midwives, and paediatricians dealing with HIV-positive babies.

19. British Paediatric Association (1988). *Report of a Working Party on AIDS in infancy and childhood.*

Glossary and abbreviations

Active immunity	Immunity acquired during life by contact with an antigen.
Adrenalin	Drug used in treatment of anaphylaxis. Amongst other actions it stimulates the heart and relaxes bronchial spasm.
Agglutinins	One type of antibody.
AIDS	Acquired Immunodeficiency Syndrome
Anaphylaxis	A severe allergic reaction characterized by collapse, shock, poor pulse, sometimes with wheezing and swelling of the soft tissues.
Anicteric	No visible jaundice. Used to describe cases of hepatitis where no jaundice can be seen.
Antibody	A blood protein which is part of the body's immunity. Antibodies are immunoglobulins and some specific types are called agglutinins.
Antigen	Any substance which can cause an immune response from the body, such as stimulating the formation of antibodies.
Anuria	Urine flow having ceased.
Apyrexial	Absence of fever (temperature under 37.5°C).
ARC	AIDS-related complex. A condition preceding AIDS.
Attack rate	See Incidence rate.
Attenuated vaccine	A live vaccine which is derived from a disease-causing organism but altered to render it harmless.
Auscultation	Listening with a stethoscope (usually to the chest).
Barrier nursing	Strict nursing in hospital with an individual room, use of masks, gowns, and gloves by all entering the room; and handwashing after contact with the patient or potentially contaminated material before attending to other patients.
BCG	Bacille Calmette–Guerin. The vaccine against tuberculosis.
BNF	British National Formulary
Booster	A term meaning a subsequent vaccination to an initial course of injections, e.g. pre-school booster, tetanus booster.

Capsulated or encapsulated bacteria	A type of bacteria with a protective capsule.
Carrier	An individual infected with an organism but without symptoms and capable of infecting others.
CDSC	Centre for Disease Surveillance and Control
CMV	Cytomegalovirus
CNS	Central nervous system
Coagulase	The ability to coagulate plasma, an index of pathogenicity in Staphylococci.
Colonization	When an organism lives in or on another living creature without being invasive or causing disease.
Commensal	An organism which normally inhabits an area without causing symptoms, e.g. *Candida* is a skin commensal.
Confluent rash	Where the spots of the rash join up.
Coryza	An acutely running nose.
CRS	Congenital rubella syndrome
CSF	Cerebrospinal fluid
DH	Department of Health (previously DHSS)
Discrete rash	A rash where the spots stay separate, cf. confluent rash.
DTP	Diphtheria/tetanus/pertussis combined vaccine
Dysentery	Diarrhoea with blood and pus (irrespective of the causative organism).
Dysuria	Pain on passing urine
EB, EBV	Epstein–Barr virus
ELISA	Enzyme-linked immunosorbent assay. A laboratory test used to diagnose a variety of diseases by detecting antibodies in blood and other body fluids.
Endemic	A disease that is always present in a community, e.g. malaria in India, measles in England.
Enteric precautions	Gloves should be used for touching contaminated materials. Hands must be washed after contact with the patient or potentially contaminated articles before contact with another person. Masks are unnecessary but gowns are needed where soiling is likely. Where possible an individual toilet facility should be used or care taken to clean a shared facility after use.
Enterotoxin	See Toxin.

Eosinophilia	A high level of a particular class of white blood cells, the eosinophils. Usually indicative of infestation or an allergic phenomenon.
Epidemic	A large-scale outbreak of disease.
Erythematous	Red appearance to skin.
Exotoxin	See Toxin.
Fatality rate	The frequency of deaths due to a disease amongst cases of the disease.
First-degree relations	For a person this includes their full brothers and sisters (siblings) and natural parents; not more distant relatives.
Fomites	Any inanimate object that may harbour a pathogenic organism, e.g. a soiled handkerchief.
HBV	Hepatitis B virus
HBVac	Vaccine against hepatitis B infection
Heaf test	One of the tests for immunity against TB.
Herd immunity	The level of immunity in the general population against a particular disease.
HIV	Human immunodeficiency virus. The cause of AIDS.
HMSO	Her Majesty's Stationery Office
Horizontal transmission	Transmission of infection from one person to another; not vertical (mother to child) transmission.
Host	An individual (human or other species) who is infected by an organism, with or without symptoms.
HRIG	Anti-rabies immunoglobulin
HSV	*Herpes simplex* virus
Hypergammaglobulinaemia	Raised gammaglobulin levels in the blood.
Hypoxia/hypoxaemia	Low levels of oxygen in the blood.
im	intramuscular
Immunity	The ability of an individual to resist disease, especially infection. Can be natural, active or passive. Natural immunity—the non-specific immunity which depends on genetic and non-specific factors (e.g. mucus secretions and antiseptic agents in sweat) and makes different species susceptible to some organisms and resistant to others. Active immunity—the specific immunity acquired by natural or induced exposure, and achieved by the immune system producing

	antibodies and cells which attack pathogens. Passive immunity—specific immunity acquired by injection of a preparation of antibodies. This also refers to the placenta from mother to fetus.
Immunization	See Vaccine.
Immunoglobulins	See Antibody.
Inactivated or killed vaccine	A vaccine made of dead material. It may be the whole organism, e.g. pertussis, or a component, e.g. pneumococcus.
Incidence rate	The number of new cases of a disease occurring in a population of defined size per unit of time.
Incubation period	The time between a person encountering an organism and symptoms appearing.
Induration	A hard area of skin or tissue.
Infancy	From birth to the first birthday.
Infection	The invasion of a host and multiplication therein by an organism. This may or may not lead to symptoms (disease).
Infectious	A disease or organism that is commonly communicated from one host (human or otherwise) to another. Contrast with diseases which are due to infectious organisms but are not communicated from one human to another, e.g. urinary-tract infections.
Intradermal injection	Immunization by injection into the layers of the skin. Used for BCG and sometimes typhoid.
ISC	Indian sub-continent
iv	intravenous
Leukocytosis	High blood white cell count.
Leukopoenia	Low blood white cell count.
Live vaccine	A vaccine made of live bacteria or virus much altered so that it is not dangerous but can still induce immunity.
Lymphadenopathy	Lymph gland enlargement.
Lymphocyte	One of the white blood cells concerned in the body's immunity.
Lymphocytosis	Unusually high number of lymphocytes.
Mantoux test	A skin test for immunity against TB.
MIG	Anti-mumps immunoglobulin
MMR	Measles, mumps, rubella combined vaccine
MOEH	Medical Officer of Environmental Health. In some areas other medical officers fulfil similar functions.
Monovalent	A vaccine with only one component, e.g. pertussis.

Morbidity rate	The amount of illness occurring amongst a defined number of people in a unit of time.
Mortality rate	The number of deaths occurring amongst a defined number of people in a unit of time.
Named-person basis	A term used to indicate that an immunization is available for use if a doctor requests it from a supplier for a particular individual, but is not yet licensed for general use. For example, this is the case for the immunization for tick-borne encephalitis (1987).
Neonate	Baby in the first 4 weeks of life.
Oliguria	Low urine output.
Parenteral	Given by injection.
Passive immunity	See Immunity.
Pathogenic	Producing disease.
Per-nasal swab	A swab used to take a sample of the mucus in a child's pharynx. It is inserted through the nostrils and is used as a test for whooping cough.
Peri-	Around. Hence perianal (around the anus), perioral (around the mouth).
Pertussis	The medical term for whooping cough.
PHLS	Public Health Laboratory Service
Primary course	Applies to diphtheria, tetanus, pertussis, and polio, and means the first three immunizations.
Proctitis	Inflammation or infection around the anus.
Prodrome	Symptoms experienced prior to the characteristic features of a specific infectious disease.
Prophylaxis	The process of protecting an individual with an agent, e.g. a vaccine or an antibiotic.
PUO	Pyrexia of unknown origin.
Pyrexia	Fever.
Pyuria	A significant number of white blood (pus) cells in the urine.
Reactogenic	An immunization producing a reaction.
Reye's syndrome	A profound illness involving liver failure and general collapse which is frequently fatal.
Rigor	A systemic reaction involving shaking associated with high fever.
Rubella	The medical term for German measles.
sc	subcutaneous
Second- and third-degree relations	Relatives more distant than brother/sister and parents, e.g. a cousin.
Serology	Looking for antibodies in an individual's blood as evidence of infection.

Seropositive and seronegative	A person whose blood shows they have antibodies (and therefore are presumed immune) to a specific disease, either because they have been immunized or have had the infection. Seronegative means not having such antibodies.
SPA	Suprapubic aspiration (of urine)
Strain	A sub-type of a species of organism, e.g. the different strains of Staphylococcus.
Subclinical	An infection where there are no overt symptoms.
Teratogenic	Producing a malformation in the fetus.
Toxin	A poison produced by an infecting organism, e.g. toxin from diphtheria or tetanus.
Toxoid	An immunization prepared from a toxin by removing its poisonous qualities but retaining its vaccinating effects, e.g. tetanus toxoid which is tetanus toxin inactivated by formaldehyde.
Triple vaccine	The immunization incorporating diphtheria, tetanus, and whooping cough (DPT).
Tympanic membrane	The ear-drum.
Vaccine	A suspension of attenuated live or killed micro-organisms or fractions thereof given to induce immunity and hence prevent infectious disease. Vaccination essentially means the same as immunization.
Vaccinee	An individual who is being immunized.
Vertical transmission	(For infectious disease) Mother-to-child transmission in the prenatal or perinatal period across the placenta, blood-borne, or via breast milk.
ZIG	Zoster immune globulin (anti-varicella immunoglobulin)

Index

Managing anaphylaxis

1. Lie the patient down on a flat surface in the left lateral position and maintain airway.
2. Check central pulses (carotid, femoral).
   (a) If pulses are STRONG, summon medical help but no '999' call needed as this is probably a faint.
   (b) If pulses are WEAK, proceed with subcutaneous or intramuscular adrenaline, apply oxygen (if available) and summon immediate assistance—call for a doctor and if necessary make an emergency call. Drug dosage intramuscular adrenalin **1:1000.**

Less than 1 year	0.05 ml im
1st to 2nd birthday	0.1 ml im
2nd to 3rd birthday	0.2 ml im
3rd to 5th birthday	0.3 ml im
5th to 6th birthday	0.4 ml im
After 6th birthday	0.5 ml im

3. If there is no improvement in the patient's condition in 10 minutes, repeat the same dose of intramuscular adrenalin.
4. If medical assistance has not arrived after 30 minutes and the patient's condition gives rise for concern, repeat the same dose of intramuscular adrenalin.
5. **A maximum of 3 doses** of adrenalin 1:1000 may be given.